Outpatient Management of Depression:
A Guide for the Primary-Care Practitioner

Second Edition

Sheldon H. Preskorn, MD

Professor and Chairman
Department of Psychiatry
University of Kansas School of Medicine

President and Medical Director
Psychiatric Research Institute
and Center for Phase I Research
Via Christi Medical Center
Wichita, Kansas

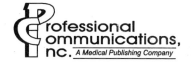

Professional
Communications,
Inc. *A Medical Publishing Company*

Published by:
Professional Communications, Inc.

For orders, please call:
1-800-337-9838

ISBN: 0-884735-46-0

Printed in the United States of America

DISCLAIMER

The opinions expressed in this publication reflect those of the author. However, the author makes no warranty regarding the contents of the publication. The protocols described herein are general and may not apply to a specific patient. Any product men-tioned in this publication should be taken in accordance with the prescribing information provided by the manufacturer.

This text is printed on recycled paper.

DEDICATION

To my wife, Belinda and daughter, Erika
with love and gratitude for your understanding,
patience and encouragement.

In memory of my parents,
Harrison and Marie Preskorn.

To Wally and Marge.

To Sister Sylvia.

To my patients.

To all of my colleagues at the
Psychiatric Research Institute and the
University of Kansas School of Medicine –
Wichita
Department of Psychiatry.

Thank you.

ACKNOWLEDGMENT

The author gratefully acknowledges Ms. Phyllis
Jones Freeny for her assistance with manuscript
preparation.

ABOUT THE AUTHOR

Sheldon H. Preskorn, MD, is a fellow of the American Psychiatric Association and the American Psychopathological Association. He has served on advisory committees of the Food and Drug Administration, Veterans Administration, National Institutes of Health and National Science Foundation, as well as consultant with the Menninger Foundation.

He received his medical degree at the University of Kansas, Kansas City, Kansas. He completed a 2-year residency in anatomical pathology (with emphasis on neuropathology) and a 1-year rotating internship in internal medicine and psychiatry at the University of Kansas Medical Center, Kansas City, Kansas. He did his residency in psychiatry at Washington University School of Medicine, St. Louis, Missouri. He has undergraduate training in psychobiology (psychology, biology and chemistry) and postgraduate medical training in anatomical pathology (neuropathology), psychiatry, and basic and clinical pharmacology.

An international lecturer and the author of 300 scientific and professional articles, Dr. Preskorn has received continuous grant funding since 1978. His principal areas of research have been in psychopharmacology, affective and anxiety disorders, and neuroscience.

His basic pharmacological and neuroscience research has included studies in learning theory, neurochemistry, neurophysiology, histochemistry, electron microscopy, cerebral blood flow and metabolism, positron emission tomography, and radioligand binding. His clinical research has included pharmacokinetics and drug development through all clinical phases, starting with "first time in man" studies through registration proceedings.

He has been the principal investigator on over 150 formal clinical trials, including drug development studies of all antidepressants marketed in the United States in the last 10 years. He has also been involved in the registration process of seven of these eight classes of drugs.

His clinical experience has included 6 years as supervising physician for an acute psychosis ward, 6 years as Chief of Psychiatry for a university-affiliated Veterans Administration Medical Center, and 7 years as Director of the Outpatient Psychiatric Clinic for the University of Kansas School of Medicine – Wichita, Kansas.

TABLE OF CONTENTS

TABLES

vii

FIGURES

Introduction

There are several major differences between the way primary-care practitioners and psychiatric physicians practice. These differences are important when considering the diagnosis and treatment of patients with major depression in the primary-care setting.[121]

Perhaps the most important difference is time. Psychiatrists will often have 60 minutes to work up a new patient while primary-care practitioners frequently have less. That time constraint is further compounded by the fact that the primary-care practitioner is often starting at an earlier stage than is the case with the psychiatrist. The primary-care practitioner must frequently consider a host of nonpsychiatric medical disorders as well as psychiatric disorders when evaluating the patient's complaints. In other instances, the primary-care practitioner may be seeing an ongoing patient who is having a first-time depressive episode. In that event, the practitioner has the benefit of having some prior knowledge of the patient but frequently has even less time scheduled for the patient visit. Of course, the fact that referrals to psychiatrists tend to be patients with more complicated and refractory disorders may more than offset any time advantage that they may appear to have. Thus, the first challenge in the primary-care or the psychiatric setting is to efficiently assess the patient and determine an initial treatment plan. A principal goal of this book is to present a way to successfully meet this challenge.

Another challenge is the recent explosion in antidepressant options available to the practicing clinician. Each year during the last decade, a new antidepressant has been marketed. While this increased array of effective antidepressants has benefited patients, it means that prescribers have more factors than ever to consider when selecting an antidepressant for a patient.

This book will provide the practitioner with:

- A basic understanding of depression
- A system for rapid diagnosis and rational and efficient management, including:
  - Patient education
  - Brief supportive counseling
  - Medication as appropriate.

In terms of treatment, this book focuses on antidepressant medications. Other effective therapies, such as formal types of psychotherapy (eg, interpersonal and cognitive behavioral), will not be discussed due to space constraints.[4,61,98] There are several useful books that deal specifically with these forms of psychotherapy that the interested reader should readily be able to find. The choice of appropriate therapy is an individual decision between patients and their clinicians.

1   **What Is Depression**

Major depression is one of the most prevalent, serious illnesses in the United States. It affects millions of people of all ages and walks of life. Although this disorder can be devastating, it is now more treatable than ever. There are now twenty-two different antidepressants belonging to one of eight pharmacologically distinct classes. Thus, major depression is to psychiatry as hypertension is to general medicine in that the clinician has a wide array of mechanistically different medications to select from when treating patients suffering from this disorder.

Since depression is a common condition that leads many patients to seek care from the primary-care practitioner, these clinicians are in the frontline of the battle against this disorder.[61,98,121] Over one-half of all patients with major depression are treated in the primary-care setting. Unfortunately, many cases go unrecognized, and those that are identified are frequently inadequately treated.[241]

There are several myths that contribute to this problem. One is the mistaken belief that major depression and other psychiatric disorders are trivial, will go away on their own, or are the result of character weakness. Another is that the treatment of these conditions is somehow mysterious such that primary-care practitioners cannot understand or treat such patients. This book will dispel these myths.

The same principles and approaches that apply to hypertension, diabetes mellitus, and other medical conditions also apply to psychiatric illnesses. Primary-care practitioners will find that the approach they use in their general-medicine practice will also apply to psychiatric illnesses. While the focus of this book is major depression, the principles discussed here are universally applicable to all psychiatric illnesses.

All diagnoses in medicine fit into one of the categories shown in Figure 1.1, arranged hierarchically from most (etiologic) to least (symptomatic) sophisticated. Critical variables in diagnosis are listed in Table 1.1.

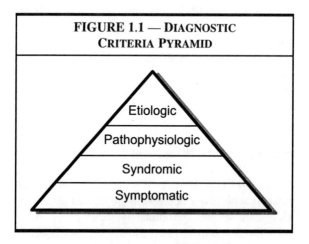

FIGURE 1.1 — DIAGNOSTIC CRITERIA PYRAMID

Etiologic
Pathophysiologic
Syndromic
Symptomatic

TABLE 1.1 — CRITICAL VARIABLES IN DIAGNOSIS

- Onset (type and age)
- Signs/symptoms
- Premorbid personality
- Family history
- Natural course
- Response to treatment
- Laboratory data

The fundamental point in diagnosing and understanding major depression is that it is a syndrome. It is not just low mood, but rather a cluster of signs and symptoms termed a depressive episode and consisting of:

- Change in mood:
  - Usually "depressed," "blue," or "sad"
  - Sometimes irritable or anxious
    (Of note, while the syndrome takes it name from the mood symptom, the two are not synonymous. Not everyone who is "blue" has major depression, nor is "depressed mood" necessarily the most prominent symptom for every patient with major depression.)
- Change in sleep patterns
- Change in appetite
- Change in weight
- Change in activity levels
- A sense of fatigue
- Decreased motivation
- Decreased interest
- Decreased sex drive
- Decreased concentration and attention.

A patient suffering from a major depressive episode will have five or more of these signs and symptoms every day for weeks to months, and even years, if not effectively treated. Diagnostic criteria for a major depressive episode as listed in the Diagnostic and Statistical Manual version IV (DSM-IV) of the American Psychiatric Association are shown in Table 1.2.

In classic or melancholic major depression, there is a decrease in:

- Sleep
- Appetite
- Weight
- Activity levels.

TABLE 1.2 — DSM-IV DIAGNOSTIC CRITERIA FOR A MAJOR DEPRESSIVE EPISODE

• Five (or more) of the following symptoms have been present during the same 2-week period and represent a change from previous functioning; at least one of the symptoms is either (1) depressed mood or (2) loss of interest or pleasure (*Note*: Do not include symptoms that are clearly due to a general medical condition, or mood-incongruent delusions or hallucinations):

– Depressed mood most of the day, nearly every day, as indicated by either subjective report (eg, feels sad or empty) or observation made by others (eg, appears tearful). *Note*: In children and adolescents, can be irritable mood

– Markedly diminished interest or pleasure in all, or almost all, activities most of the day, nearly every day (as indicated by either subjective account or observation made by others)

– Significant weight loss when not dieting or weight gain (eg, a change of more than 5% of body weight in a month), or decrease or increase in appetite nearly every day. Note: In children, consider failure to make expected weight gains

– Insomnia or hypersomnia nearly every day

– Psychomotor agitation or retardation nearly every day (observable by others, not merely subjective feelings of restlessness or being slowed down)

– Fatigue or loss of energy nearly every day

– Feelings of worthlessness or excessive or inappropriate guilt (which may be delusional) nearly every day (not merely self-reproach or guilt about being sick)

– Diminished ability to think or concentrate; indecisiveness, nearly every day (either by subjective account or as observed by others)

– Recurrent thoughts of death (not just fear of dying), recurrent suicidal ideation without a specific plan, or a suicide attempt or a specific plan for committing suicide

- The symptoms do not meet criteria for a mixed episode
- The symptoms cause clinically significant distress or impairment in social, occupational, or other important areas of functioning
- The symptoms are not due to the direct physiological effects of a substance (eg, a drug of abuse, a medication) or a general medical condition (eg, hypothyroidism)
- The symptoms are not better accounted for by bereavement, ie, after the loss of a loved one; the symptoms persist for longer than 2 months or are characterized by marked functional impairment, morbid preoccupation with worthlessness, suicidal ideation, psychotic symptoms, or psychomotor retardation

Adapted from: *DSM-IV: Diagnostic and Statistical Manual of Mental Disorders.* 4th ed. Washington, DC: American Psychiatric Press; 1994.

However, there is also an "atypical" or "reversed vegetative symptom" syndrome in which these symptoms are increased (Table 1.3):

- Hypersomnolence
- Hyperphagia
- Weight gain
- Lethargy
- Agitation.

This atypical form has an earlier age of onset (late teens to late twenties) compared to the melancholic form (late thirties to late forties). The atypical form also has a unique family pattern: female relatives with atypical major depression and male relatives with alcoholism. In contrast, the family pattern in the melancholic form tends to be more one of pure major depression. These differences suggest that these are different forms of clinical depression. There are also some data to suggest a differential response to differ-

TABLE 1.3 — SIGNS AND SYMPTOMS OF DIFFERENT TYPES OF AFFECTIVE EPISODES

Sign/Symptom	Melancholia	Atypical or Nonclassic Depression	Hypomania
Mood	Depressed Anxious Irritable	Irritable Anxious Depressed	Irritable Euphoric
Affect	↓ Reactivity	↑ Reactivity	↑ Reactivity
Energy (subjective)	↓	↓	↑
Activity (objective)	↓	↑	↑
Sleep	↓	↑	↓
Appetite	↓	↑	↓
Sex drive	↓	↓	↑
Concentration/ attention	↓	↓	↓
Interest	↓	↓	↑

ent classes of antidepressants in patients with melancholic versus atypical clinical depression (Chapter 8).

The diagnosis of major depression can be compared to the diagnosis of migraine. A patient presents with a symptom, such as low mood in the case of major depression or headache in the case of migraine. The clinician then screens the patient for the syndrome. A pathophysiological cause, perhaps hypothyroidism in the case of a depressive syndrome or increased intracranial pressure in the case of migrainous-like headache, is checked. The clinician then should go on to explore possible etiological causes.

Major depression is currently at the syndromic level of understanding, but research is expanding our knowledge at the levels of pathophysiology and etiology, just as with any medical condition. The clinician, when faced with a patient who may have a depressive syndrome, must do differential diagnosis to confirm the diagnosis or find another explanation.

The most common known etiologies of a depressive episode include:

- Substance abuse and/or dependence involving:
  - Sedatives, especially alcohol
  - Stimulants, especially cocaine
- Other drug therapy, such as antihypertensives, particularly those that antagonize central biogenic amine mechanisms (ie, norepinephrine, serotonin, and dopamine)
- Occult malignancies:
  - Should be thoroughly considered when:
    - Patient is in high-risk group (eg, elderly)
    - Weight loss is out of proportion to other depressive symptoms
    - The depressive episode remains refractory despite adequate trials of several classes of antidepressants and/or electroconvulsive therapy (ECT)
  - A classic scenario is carcinoma of the head or the pancreas.

It is necessary to consider these common medical causes of a depressive episode because they require different treatments.

The bottom line is that clinical or major depression is a syndromic diagnosis made after excluding other medical conditions.

Once the diagnosis has been made, the clinician should endeavor to determine whether the patient has manic-depressive (also called bipolar) disorder or unipolar major depression. In bipolar illness, the patient is susceptible to hypomanic or manic episodes (Table 1.3) as well as depressive episodes, while in the latter the patient only has depressive episodes. The uni-

17

polar condition is considerably more common—about 10 times more prevalent—than the bipolar form. Nonetheless, some patients with manic-depressive illness will present for the first time with a depressive episode rather than a manic episode. It is important to make this distinction because bipolar patients are at risk for the development of a manic episode during treatment of their depressive episode (Chapter 11). If the clinician is alert to this possibility, steps can be taken (eg, concomitant treatment with lithium and increased vigilance) to decrease the risk associated with a switch into mania.

The question is how to determine whether the patient has a bipolar rather than a unipolar disorder? That can be more difficult than it may first appear. The problem is not with mania since the psychosis and/or level of functional impairment due to overt mania is such that even a casual observer can detect the condition. The problem is with hypomanic episodes. The symptoms involve the same functions as those found in major depression (Table 1.3) but differ in their expression (eg, increased rather than decreased activity) or are experienced differently (eg, the depressed patient complains of "not being able to sleep" while the hypomanic patient reports "not needing to sleep"). Rarely, if ever, do hypomanic patients present complaining about hypomania (eg, "Gee, Doc, I feel too good."). Hence, the clinician must inquire about such episodes in all patients presenting with a first-time episode of major depression.

The family history can also be helpful. Bipolar disorder has one of the strongest, if not the strongest, familial patterns of any psychiatric illness. If one or more of the patient's first- or second-degree family relatives has bipolar disorder, the clinician should consider the patient to be at increased risk, and may wish either to treat with lithium in addition to an antidepressant (Chapter 11) or instruct the patient to con-

18

tact the clinician if s/he should begin feeling "too good," "wound up," or having one of the other symptoms listed in Table 1.3.

In summary, *to make a diagnosis of a major depression, the clinician must first establish that the patient has a depressive episode and, second, rule out known medical causes of such episodes.*

2   Why Identify and Treat Major Depression

The number of people in the United States with major depression is estimated to be between 5% and 11% of the total population.[4,61,98] Over half of these individuals will have recurrent episodes periodically throughout their lives (Table 2.1). In terms of the associated mortality, morbidity, and societal costs, the impact of clinical depression is astounding (Table 2.2).

The cost to American society of depressive disorders is estimated to be $26 billion annually. This estimate does not include the effect of depression on the family.

Forty thousand to 50,000 Americans die annually because of suicide (Table 2.3). Suicide is the seventh leading cause of death in the United States. Of patients with untreated recurrent major depression, 15% will die of suicide. In up to 70% of these cases, clinical depression will be the proximal cause of death. These figures place clinical depression in the same league as leukemia as a cause of death in the United States. Suicide is the third leading cause of death among teenagers and young adults. Suicide also has an impact on the lives of the relatives, friends, and coworkers of the suicide victim. Deaths also occur as a result of accidents caused by the impaired concentration and attention characteristic of major depression.

Having major depression also increases the risk of alcohol abuse and cigarette smoking. These conditions in turn increase health problems.

Patients with major depression frequently self-medicate with alcohol to help themselves sleep and/or to reduce associated anxiety. Tragically, alcohol

TABLE 2.1 — UNIPOLAR DEPRESSION IN THE UNITED STATES

- High rate of occurrence:
  - 5% to 11% lifetime prevalence
  - 10 to 14 million in the United States depressed in any year[259]
- Episodes can be of long duration (years)
- 50% rate of recurrence following a single episode; higher if patient has had multiple episodes or a positive family history
- Morbidity comparable to angina and advanced coronary artery disease
- High mortality from suicide if untreated

TABLE 2.2 — THE HIDDEN COST OF NOT TREATING MAJOR DEPRESSION

Mortality
- 30,000 to 35,000 suicides per year[103]
- Fatal accidents due to impaired concentration and attention
- Death due to illnesses which can be a sequelae (eg, alcohol abuse)

Patient Morbidity
- Suicide attempts
- Accidents
- Resultant illnesses
- Lost jobs
- Failure to advance in career and school
- Substance abuse

Societal Costs
- Dysfunctional families
- Absenteeism
- Decreased productivity
- Job-related injuries
- Adverse effect on quality control in the workplace

TABLE 2.3 — SUICIDE AND MAJOR DEPRESSION: THE RULE OF SEVEN

- One out of seven people with recurrent depressive illness commit suicide[72]
- Seventy percent of suicides have depressive illness[206]
- Seventy percent of suicides see their primary-care practitioner within 6 weeks of suicide[207]
- Suicide is the seventh leading cause of death in the United States[103]

provides only fleeting relief and then aggravates the underlying biochemistry of clinical depression, setting up the potential for a downward, vicious spiral.

The incidence of cigarette smoking is higher in depressed individuals and may be a harder habit to break in this population. In a prospective study of almost 3,000 patients, depression was found to be associated with a 5 times greater number of disability days in employed individuals. Other studies have found depression to be associated with:

- Poorer physical health
- Increased health-care utilization.

Based on a 15-year prospective outcome study, 80% of depressed individuals who are not treated will have a poor outcome, either remaining ill or experiencing recurrence(s) of their illness. The disability due to major depression is on par with or worse than that of chronic medical illnesses such as coronary artery disease, hypertension, diabetes mellitus, and arthritis, adversely affecting:

- Health-care utilization
- Absenteeism at work
- Productivity
- Job-related injuries
- Quality control in the workplace due to impaired concentration and attention.

To fully appreciate the impact of depression, the following would also have to be quantified:

- The cost of decreased work productivity by depressed individuals suffering functional impairment due to major depression
- The impact on the individual and their family of:
  - Failure to advance in one's education
  - Failure to advance in one's career
  - Lost jobs
  - Marital strife
  - Family dysfunction.

Major depression (Table 2.4):

- Is twice as likely to occur in women
- Has a peak age of onset from 20 to 40 years of age
- Runs in families—if there is a family history of major depression, a person has a three-fold higher likelihood of developing this disorder in comparison to the general population
- Has a greater incidence among separated and divorced people (which is cause versus which is effect is not known, since major depression may cause separation and divorce)
- Is more likely to be reported in unmarried than married men (again, the causal relationship is unclear)
- Is more likely to be reported in married than unmarried women (again, the causal relationship is unknown since depressed women with chronic low self-esteem may settle for abusive and dysfunctional mates)
- Has an increased risk of occurrence for women during the last trimester, the first 6 months following childbirth, and during the onset of menopause as well as an increase in symptoms prior to menses (suggesting a possible role for

TABLE 2.4 — RISK FACTORS FOR MAJOR DEPRESSION

Risk Factor	Association
Gender	Major depression is twice as likely in women
Age	Peak age of onset is 20 to 40 years of age
Family history	3 times higher risk with positive history
Marital status	Separated and divorced persons report higher rates
	Married males lower rates than unmarried males
	Married females higher rates than unmarried females
Postpartum	An increased risk for the 6-month period following childbirth
Negative life events	Possible association
Early parental death	Possible association

fluctuations in sex hormones as pathophysiologically important "triggers" for the expression of the illness). Of interest, neuronal systems (norepinephrine and serotonin) that have been implicated in the pathophysiology of the illness are influenced by fluctuations in estrogen levels.

Women are more likely to experience a depressive episode, while men are more likely to suffer from alcohol abuse and dependence. In fact, a subset of males who abuse alcohol may do so because of having undetected major depression. Effective treatment of their alcoholism may require concomitant treatment of their depressive illness.

Fortunately, advances have been made in the understanding of what constitutes appropriate and effective treatment, such as:

- The development of eight pharmacologically unique classes of antidepressants with varying spectra of antidepressant activity (Chapters 6 through 8)
- Better definition of what constitutes a therapeutic trial of an antidepressant in terms of dose and duration (Chapter 9)
- An enhanced knowledge of clinically meaningful pharmacokinetics and pharmacodynamics to increase the safety and efficacy of these antidepressants (Chapters 6 and 10).

As a result of these developments, the prognosis of clinical depression is among the best of any major medical illness. Approximately 50% of patients with major depression fully remit when treated with any antidepressant. Of the remaining 50%, the majority will respond to monodrug treatment with an antidepressant from a mechanistically different class (Chapters 6 through 8).

Tragically, many patients are not treated.[241] In one study, only 3.5% of over 6,000 cases of newly diagnosed depressed patients had received appropriate antidepressant treatment (eg, dose, duration). Hence, many "treatment refractory" cases are actually cases of inadequate treatment.

3 How to Establish the Diagnosis in the Primary-Care Setting

A challenge for the primary-care practitioner is how to efficiently and accurately determine whether a patient is suffering from major depression alone or in combination with a comorbid medical illness (eg, a patient with diabetes mellitus who is also suffering from major depression). This task is even more challenging because there are no confirmatory or screening laboratory tests that are sufficiently sensitive or specific to be clinically useful. Thus, the diagnosis must be based on clinical grounds:

- Medical history
- Physical examination
- Laboratory tests; to rule out other medical conditions that can cause a depressive episode.

The primary presenting picture generally falls into one of four categories:

- Mood or emotional complaints:
  - Low self-esteem or feelings of inadequacy
  - Anxiety
  - Irritability
  - Apathy
  - Loss of interest
- Somatic complaints:
  - Insomnia
  - Fatigue
  - Headache
  - Weight change (loss or gain)
- "Memory" problems

- Life complaints:
  - Inability to cope with marital or job stresses
  - Social withdrawal or isolation
  - Financial problems.

The clinician may unfortunately conclude that the depressive symptoms are understandable results of the patient's life situation and/or recent stressors. While that connection may seem obvious given cultural beliefs, it is often wrong. Major depression may be the *cause* of the life problems rather than being the *result* of them. After all, this illness can adversely affect work performance, motivation, and social skills.

Having a "reason" for major depression does not alter its course, reduce its severity and consequences, nor change its responsiveness to treatment. Nonetheless, clinicians may not treat major depression if they perceive that the patient "has a reason for being depressed." However, they would never think of not treating a myocardial infarction or lung carcinoma because the patient has a "reason" for having the illness, such as being overweight or being a smoker, respectively.

Further complicating the diagnostic process is the fact that some patients will deny the mood symptoms of clinical depression, yet present with all the other symptoms (Figure 3.1).

What to Do After the Suspicion of Major Depression Has Arisen

There are many possible medical causes of a depressive episode, which need to be efficiently assessed and ruled out to arrive at a diagnosis of major depression. The diagnostic process can be accomplished by following these steps:

STEP 1. Establish whether a depressive syndrome is present based on eliciting the requisite signs and symptoms (Table 1.3). While there may be some fluctuation in the symptom severity throughout the day or from day to day, the symptoms should be present every day for a minimum of 2 weeks. The longer the duration of the depressive syndrome, the less likely it will spontaneously remit. Based on clinical trials research, depressive episodes that have lasted for more than 3 months are unlikely to spontaneously abate or respond to placebo.

STEP 2. While time is of the essence in the primary-care setting, the confidence in the diagnosis is higher if the patient reports the depressive syndrome with as little prompting as possible by the clinician. For this reason, it is preferable not to immediately go to a litany of yes-no questions such as "have you been having trouble falling to sleep at night?"

The following series of hierarchically arranged questions is recommended to establish the presence of a depressive episode:

■ **Question 1**

You have been having problems with [use patient's words] (eg, "depression," "insomnia," "stress at work"). What else have you noticed about how you have been feeling or acting?

This question is phrased to elicit as many spontaneous reports of the signs and symptoms of a depressive episode as possible. The clinician can then follow-up and clarify the patient's answer(s) in terms

FIGURE 3.1 — DIAGNOSTIC AND TREATMENT PLANNING PROCESS

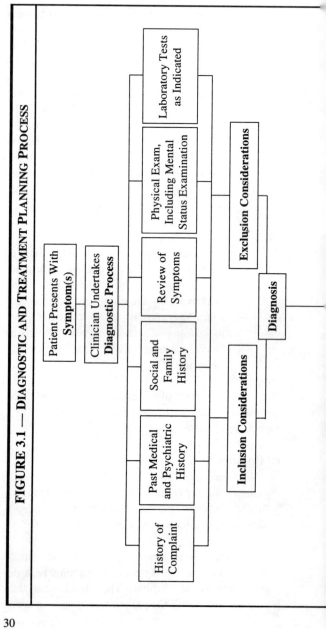

30

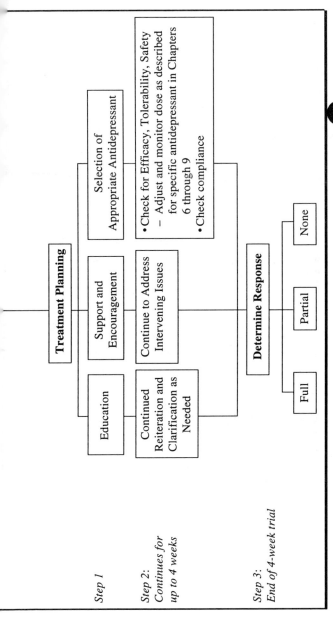

Treatment Planning

Education	Support and Encouragement	Selection of Appropriate Antidepressant
Continued Reiteration and Clarification as Needed	Continue to Address Intervening Issues	• Check for Efficacy, Tolerability, Safety – Adjust and monitor dose as described for specific antidepressant in Chapters 6 through 9 • Check compliance

Determine Response

Full	Partial	None

Step 1

Step 2:
Continues for
up to 4 weeks

Step 3:
End of 4-week trial

31

of duration, clustering, temporal stability, and severity. Frequently, a patient who presents with mood or emotional symptoms will remain fixed on these complaints when asked Question 1. In this case, the clinician can move to the next more focused question.

■ Question 2

I understand that you have been feeling [using patient's words] (eg, "depressed," "sad," "hopeless," "overwhelmed"). Has this affected you physically?

This question is designed to shift the patient's mental set to somatic signs and symptoms of major depression (ie, sleep, appetite, energy, activity, sex drive, and concentration/attention). The patient who has major depression will generally report a number of these symptoms at this point. At that point, the clinician can explore duration, clustering, temporal stability, and severity. Based on the answers to this series of questions, the clinician will have gathered sufficient data to have a reasonable opinion as to whether the patient is experiencing a depressive episode. To completely and fully assess the severity of the syndrome, the clinician can then move to highly specific questions, such as:

■ Question 3

Since you have been [using patient's words] (eg, "depressed," "bothered by headaches"), have you also been having problems with:
- *Mood (being depressed, irritable, anxious)*
- *Sleep (too little or too much)*
- *Appetite (too little or too much)*
- *Energy (subjective)*
- *Activity (objective)*
- *Interest*
- *Motivation*

- *Concentration/attention*
- *Sex drive.*

If desired, this portion can also be done by having the patient complete a checklist or by having appropriate clinic staff (eg, office nurse) conduct this portion of the interview. If any answers to the questions on this list are positive and represent new findings, further questions may be needed to assess their duration, temporal stability, and severity, and whether they have occurred as a cluster with any other previously elicited depressive symptoms.

By using these three questions, the clinician can evaluate whether the patient fulfills criteria for a depressive syndrome. Most often, the diagnosis will be major depression. Nonetheless, a depressive syndrome can be due to several other causes. Hence, the clinician needs to rule out other possibilities.

Work-Up for Other Causes of a Depressive Syndrome

(Table 3.1)
- Medical history and physical examination—the clinician can assess for a variety of other medical causes of major depression
- History of present illness—be alert for any signs of symptoms that are not typically associated with major depression (eg, productive cough)
- Past medical history—are there any past illnesses that could be recurrent and cause a depressive syndrome?
- Medications—is the patient taking any medications (eg, antihypertensives, steroids) which could cause a depressive syndrome?
- Social history—is the patient drinking alcohol or abusing illicit drugs?

TABLE 3.1 — TYPICAL BEHAVIOR DURING OFFICE VISIT

Behavior	Depressed Patient	Not Depressed Patient
Affect	• Sad/anxious affect • Sad/anxious expressions • Stooped, sagging posture • Frequent negative statements	• Predominantly positive affect • Full range of affective expressions • Facial animation • Frequent positive and affect-laden expressions
Rate of behavior	• Decreased rate of behavior • Speaks less often • Speaks with less intensity • Looks at others less • Less spontaneous	• Sustained, spontaneous, and appropriate goal-directed behavior
Responsiveness	• Responses slow and halting • Frequent nonacknowledgment • Sadness and withdrawal in response to anger or irritation in others • Critical of others	• Normal rate and rhythm of response • Responses affectively appropriate

Tolerance	• Frequently irritable/hostile, especially in intimate relationships • Low stress tolerance • Irritability increases as stress increases	• Normal stress tolerance
Adaptation to stressful situations (eg, work, home)	• Uses strategies requiring least cognitive effort • Forced obedience • Withdrawal in face of resistance • Benign neglect	• Able to negotiate solutions • Attentive to behavior and contingent responses • Able to foster sustained positive interactions

- Family history—are there other family members with major depression or other psychiatric disorders that could be presenting as a depressive syndrome? Remember most psychiatric illnesses run in families. The family history therefore can help elucidate and support the diagnosis. Conditions such as somatization disorder (eg, Briquet's syndrome) can present with waxing and waning complaints of dysphoria and anxiety and lead to a false-positive diagnosis of major depression. Somatization disorders tend to run in families, so check whether other relatives (particularly females) have complicated medical histories. A family history of bipolar disorder increases the likelihood that the patient will eventually have a manic episode, and treatment with a mood stabilizer (eg, lithium) might be warranted, either alone or in combination with an antidepressant (Chapter 11).
- Physical observation—the patient with major depression typically will have the following findings (Figure 3.1 and Table 3.2):
  - Diminished eye contact
  - Sad, apathetic, or emotionally blunted expression
  - Stooped posture
  - Decreased rate and rhythm of speech
  - Increased latency of response.

  Less often, patients will show:
  - Irritability
  - Psychomotor restlessness (eg, drumming fingers, biting nails). The efficient clinician can assess the mental status while obtaining the history and will also be comparing the patient's subjective statements about the severity of the patient's condition with observations of behavior during the interview.

TABLE 3.2 — VARIED TERMS USED FOR DEPRESSED MOOD	
Depressed Person May Report Being:	**Others May Describe the Depressed Person as Being:**
Down	Gloomy
Sad	Pessimistic
Unhappy	Cynical
Discouraged	Grim
Empty	Negative
Miserable	Moody
Beaten	Serious
Defeated	Stern
Hopeless	Severe
Helpless	Oppressive

- Laboratory tests—the standard laboratory work-up is to evaluate other possible medical causes. These tests include:
  - Complete blood cell count
  - Liver, renal, and thyroid function tests *AST ALT BUN CR TSH*
  - Urinalysis
  - Serology for infectious diseases (if the history warrants). Other laboratory tests would be more patient specific, such as an electrocardiogram, depending on the age of the patient, or brain imaging if a neurological condition needs to be assessed.

For the primary-care clinician who has treated the patient for some time, the above history may either already be known or can be quickly elicited. If that is not the case, then the clinician or a staff member can obtain that information at either the initial or a follow-up visit. That decision should be based on the clinician's assessment of how likely it is that this information would substantially alert his/her opinion and course of treatment.

Note: The above has focused on differential diagnosis and thus has discussed major depression and other medical conditions from an "either/or" perspective. In fact, clinical depression is frequently comorbid with a variety of other medical illnesses (eg, cancer, diabetes, coronary artery disease). In such instances, both conditions need to be treated for optimal outcome. Otherwise, untreated clinical depression can seriously compromise the ability to effectively treat the whole patient. This fact also means the clinician needs to be mindful of the potential for interactions between the various medications the patient will be taking. This issue and its relevance to antidepressant drug selection is discussed in greater detail in Chapters 6 and 10.

To Treat or Not to Treat Now?

If the severity of the syndrome is mild and/or not convincingly present, the clinician may decide to defer initiating antidepressant pharmacotherapy and schedule the patient for a follow-up within 1 week. This approach permits an assessment of the temporal stability of the patient's complaints. That is particularly true if somatization disorder is suspected because depressive and anxiety complaints in such patients may be prominent one week and gone the next.

Conversely, if the illness is sufficiently severe to be causing distress and/or dysfunction, the prescriber may elect to start a trial of medication, and schedule a follow-up visit in 1 week. Chapters 6 through 9 provide a way of evaluating which antidepressant is likely to be the best option for a specific patient.

4 What to Say to the Depressed Patient and How to Say It

As part of the treatment planning, the clinician must decide whether to treat the patient as an outpatient, in the hospital, or refer to a psychiatrist. Hospitalization is generally based on the following considerations:

- Is the patient at high risk for suicide?
- Is the patient psychotic?
- Is the patient so functionally impaired that s/he cannot ensure that basic needs will be met?

How to Assess the Suicide Risk

The prediction of suicide risk is imperfect at best, although often obvious in hindsight. There are risk factors that can be useful when assessing the patient's potential for suicide (Table 4.1).

Previous suicide attempts bear special comment since they are counterintuitive. Patients can be divided into those who have a history of no or one previous suicide attempt and those with multiple suicide attempts (more than 4 previous attempts). The latter history is more suggestive of a personality disorder rather than major depression. Such patients are more at risk for future attempts than for suicide completion. While it may initially seem counterintuitive, the absence of a history of previous attempts does not substantially diminish the risk of suicide completion. The reason is that the majority of patients who commit suicide do so on their first or second attempt. When the clinician is confronted with a moderate to more se-

TABLE 4.1 — RISK FACTORS FOR SUICIDE: "SAD PERSONS" SCALE

S — *Sex*: More than three males for every one female kill themselves[206]

A — *Age*: Older > younger, especially Caucasian males

D — *Depression*: A depressive episode precedes suicide in up to 70% of cases

P — *Previous attempt(s)*: Most people who die from suicide do so on their first or second attempt. Patients who make multiple (4+) attempts have increased risk of future attempts rather than suicide completion

E — *Ethanol use*: Recent onset of ethanol or other sedative-hypnotic drug use increases the risk and may be a form of self medication

R — *Rational thinking loss*: Profound cognitive slowing, psychotic depression, pre-existing brain damage, particularly frontal lobes

S — *Social support deficit*: May be result of the illness which can cause social withdrawal

O — *Organized plan*: Always need to inquire about presence of a plan when treating a depressed patient

N — *No spouse*: Again, may be a result rather than a cause of the depressive disorder, but nevertheless absence of a spouse or significant other is a risk factor

S — *Sickness*: Intercurrent medical illnesses

vere, full depressive syndrome in a previously nonaffected, middle-age-to-older patient, then suicide risk must be carefully considered regardless of whether s/he has made a previous attempt. This issue is particularly important in the patient who has:

- A positive family history for suicide
- Prominent feelings of hopelessness and/or guilt.

How to Inquire About Suicidal Ideation

Some clinicians are uncomfortable about inquiring about suicidal ideation. They believe that it will anger the patient. Others believe that it may "plant the seed." A few may not want to know the answer.

The first two concerns can be easily dispelled. Most patients will be relieved and thankful that the clinician was sufficiently concerned to inquire, assuming it is done in a tactful manner as discussed below. There is also no evidence that such questioning prompts patients to commit suicide. Instead, it uncovers patients at risk so that appropriate preventive steps can be taken.

At the time the patient describes a depressive episode, the clinician can empathize with the patient and simultaneously begin exploring for the presence of suicidal ideation by saying:

"You sound as if you have been feeling pretty miserable. Has life ever seemed not worth living?"

In response, most patients will spontaneously state they have or have not had such thoughts. They often will go on to say that they would never commit suicide for a variety of reasons (eg, religious beliefs, effect on family and friends). If the patient acknowledges feeling that s/he would be better off dead, but does not explicitly state how actively s/he has contemplated suicide, the clinician can follow-up by asking:

"So, you have felt that life was not worth living. Have you ever thought about acting on those feelings?"

If the patient acknowledges that s/he has, the clinician should then explore how far such thinking has gone:

- Does s/he have a plan?
- If so, what is it?

- Has s/he acted on it?
- If so, how recently?

If the patient has made a plan, has the means, or has recently acted on it, then hospitalization is obviously needed. If the patient is in a gray area, the clinician must decide how impulsive the patient is and whether a good faith agreement can be made to contact the clinician or come to a care facility if suicidal ideation becomes intrusive, persistent, and compelling.

Is the Patient Psychotic?

A small percentage of patients with major depression in the primary-care setting will have a mood-congruent hallucination or delusion. Examples include: the patient hears a voice stating that s/he is evil and deserves to die, or the patient believes that s/he has contracted a serious illness as a punishment for an earlier imaged sin or transgression. Such patients warrant hospitalization because of the likelihood of acting on the psychosis.

Is the Episode So Severe That Hospitalization Is Necessary?

This issue requires the clinician to make several assessments:

- How much functional impairment has the depressive episode caused?
- What are the functional demands on the patient at work and at home?
- Are there support systems that can help offset any imbalance between the patient's functional status and the functional demands on the patient?

Based on the answers to the questions, the clinician can determine whether the patient needs a release from work and needs further functional support, up to and including hospitalization.

Most patients with major depression seen in a primary-care setting can be appropriately treated on an outpatient basis. Nonetheless, the decision of where to treat and whether to seek a consult or refer must be made with careful deliberation.

4

Initiating Outpatient Therapy

The first step is educational and empathic counseling. Patients with any illness present with questions outlined in Table 4.2. Added to these universal questions are the following issues commonly encountered in patients with major depression:

- They feel guilty or responsible for their illness
- In searching for a reason, they often attribute their illness to outside factors such as "stresses" on the job or at home
- Job or home-life problems may be a result rather than a cause of their illness.

The clinician and staff need to address these issues empathically and efficiently. That can be done

---

TABLE 4.2 — PATIENT'S TYPICAL QUESTIONS ABOUT MAJOR DEPRESSION

- What do I have?
- Will I feel better?
- What will it take to feel better?
- What should I do?
- What should I not do?
- Will it happen again?
- Do I need to be on medications indefinitely?
- Why did this happen to me?

by anticipating common issues and providing standard educational information without having to wait for the patient to ask. The common questions/issues that patients have include:

■ What Do I Have?

You have major depression. Like many illnesses, we do not completely know what causes it. We do know that it runs in families like other illnesses such as diabetes and hypertension. That fact and others lead us to believe that major depression is due to biochemical changes in brain function, sometimes described as a "chemical imbalance."

Although many patients who are depressed think they caused it or that it is a sign of personal weakness, there is no evidence to support this belief. It is no more true for major depression than for diabetes or hypertension.

■ Will I Feel Better?

Yes. While we do not know precisely what causes major depression, we do have a number of effective treatments for it. With such treatment, you have an excellent chance of being over this episode in a matter of weeks. Without such treatment, you might get better spontaneously, but it could take months or even years. Unfortunately, antidepressants do not work for depressive episodes as aspirins do for headaches. It may take 2 to 4 weeks of treatment before you start to notice substantial improvement. Nonetheless, *you will begin to feel better.*

You can think of response to antidepressants like the treatment of a sore throat with antibiotics. While the antibiotic begins to kill the bacteria within hours of starting it, there is a period before you notice the improvement. In the case of antibiotics, the delay is a couple of days. With antidepressants, it may be a couple of weeks. Bear with it because you will begin to feel better.

In the case of both antibiotics and antidepressants, you should continue treatment for a period even after you feel better. We generally advise you to keep taking an antibiotic for 5 to 7 days after you feel better to ensure complete eradication of the bacteria and thus reduce the likelihood of a recurrence of the infection. We advise that you continue taking an antidepressant for 4 to 5 more months after you feel better because that is the interval during which you are at risk for a relapse. We will discuss this issue further after you are feeling better. The point now is to get you well.

■ What Will It Take to Feel Better?

We use *antidepressant medications to shorten the time necessary to get over an episode.* Most patients will experience either *significant improvement or a full remission from their episode within a couple of weeks* of starting an antidepressant. In some individuals, full improvement can take 6 to 8 weeks. Remember that these medications take time to work and do not be discouraged by the fact that you do not feel immediate relief. For you to respond, you need to take the medication regularly as prescribed.

Some patients may worry that others might think that taking antidepressant medication is a sign of "weakness." People would never accuse a patient with diabetes of being weak for taking insulin. You are feeling badly enough and you should not be berating yourself for your illness. Instead, let us work together to get you well.

Some patients wonder whether medications are the total answer. They virtually never are for any significant illness, whether it is major depression or hypertension. At a minimum, you need to know about the illness so that you can optimally deal with it.

Many patients with major depression will respond fully to supportive counseling plus medications Others may need more formal counseling called psychotherapy. Generally, that decision is an individual one, between the clinician and the patient.

■ What Should I Do?

There are several steps you can take to help in your treatment. It is important to *learn about your condition* so that you will know what to expect, particularly during the initial period of treatment. *Do not blame yourself* for your major depression. Realize that you did not ask to suffer from it. Your self-esteem has likely been shaken as would be true for anyone who has had such an episode. *Give yourself a reprieve from negative thinking* for now. Take your medication as prescribed. Get plenty of rest, stay physically active, eat regularly, and keep socially involved.

■ What Should I Not Do?

Do not drink alcohol when suffering from major depression. Alcohol causes similar changes in brain chemistry as occurs during a depressive episode. Many patients with major depression attempt to self-medicate by drinking alcohol to either help themselves sleep or to "calm their nerves." Don't do it. While it may initially help you to fall asleep, its sedative effect wears off quickly causing early morning awakening. For the same reason, do not use illicit drugs, or other sedative agents or stimulants.

Do not make any major life decisions while moderately or more severely depressed. What may seem like a mountain of a problem when you are feeling poorly may seem much more manageable when you are feeling better.

■ Will It Happen Again?

Although the focus now should be on getting well, you may be concerned about the risk of future episodes. The risk is primarily dependent on three factors: the duration of the current episode, the number of previous episodes, and your family history of major depression.

The likelihood of having recurrent episodes increases if your first episode has lasted longer than 2 years, which is one compelling reason to treat it aggressively now. Your risk also increases with each subsequent episode (70% with one previous episode, 90% with two previous episodes) and with each first-degree relative (parents, siblings, offspring) who suffers from major depression.[61]

The important thing is that *major depression is highly treatable.* The vast majority of patients respond to antidepressant medications. Most respond to the first agent used, but some require treatment with a second antidepressant. Unfortunately, we cannot "culture the bug" that causes major depression like we can with a sore throat. If we could, we would be able to select precisely the medication that would treat your depressive episode the first time every time. Since we cannot do that yet, we choose the medication that we think is most likely to help you. If you do not respond to it, then we will use a different type of antidepressant. Approximately, 60% of patients will respond to the first medication.[103] Of the 40% who do not, the majority will respond to the other antidepressants, bringing the overall likelihood of response to approximately 90%.

As you can see, *major depression, if treated, has an excellent prognosis* and *you should be feeling better soon.*

■ Do I Need to Be on Medications Indefinitely?

For the vast majority of patients, the answer is *no.* For first-time episodes, we will treat you for 4 to 5 months after you respond (total of 6 months of therapy) and up to 12 months or longer for recurrent episodes. After that period, we will taper and discontinue the medication. (*Note*: Some researchers advise indefinite therapy if the patient has had three previous episodes.)

We will educate you about the early signs of a recurrent episode when we taper the medication. If you should have a recurrence, this education can help you identify it early and come back for treatment before the episode fully develops.

Some people with recurrent episodes may go years between episodes so that prophylactic therapy with antidepressants does not seem to be reasonable; instead each episode is treated individually, much like recurrent episodes of a sore throat. *Although antidepressant medications have been used to prevent recurrent episodes as well as to treat existing episodes,* the decision to stay on medication to prevent future episodes is your decision. After all, you are the one who has to put up with the cost of treatment and any adverse effects that the medication may cause. Generally the decision to go on maintenance therapy is made *when the episodes become frequent and/or severe.* We do not need to make those decisions now and will discuss it more after you have been well for several months.

■ Why Did This Happen to Me?

No one completely understands why some people suffer from major depression, although it is clear that *patients do not cause or wish themselves to get ill.* As we mentioned, the condition runs in families, suggesting an inherited susceptibility. We can think of clinical depression much like any other medical illness such as diabetes or high blood pressure. Medication plays a vital role in restoring normal body function. You play an important role in your recovery by understanding your condition to the best of your ability and by *taking an active and committed role in your recovery.*

5 When to Institute Antidepressant Drug Therapy

If the patient has been evaluated, the diagnosis of major depression confirmed, and the current episode is causing considerable pain and functional impairment (but not so severe as to necessitate hospitalization), the first step is to provide education and support regarding major depression. Then, the question becomes whether to recommend antidepressant medication.

From this author's perspective, the clinician's role should be that of an advisor to the patient, as opposed to dictating any particular treatment plan. Following this philosophy, the clinician should properly assess the patient's complaints and give sufficient information about treatment options so the patient can make an informed decision on his/her own behalf. In the instance where the patient is unable to make such a decision, there are procedural steps (eg, commitment) to follow to ensure that the patient receives proper medical attention; however, that issue is beyond the scope of this book.

The patient may not select the option that the clinician feels is most appropriate. The question then is whether the clinician is comfortable with the patient's choice. If not, further discussion should be pursued or the patient should be referred to a psychiatrist. The underlying philosophy is that the patient should play an active role in the treatment planning. Often, patients will defer to a clinician's judgment, but that is their decision.

This patient-oriented approach has several advantages over a clinician simply telling the patient what needs to be done. Serious illness, such as major depression, often diminishes the patient's self-esteem and confidence. The patient-oriented approach enhances the patient's self-esteem by implicitly communicating to the patient that the clinician values the patient's judgment and wishes. Compliance with the treatment plan is also enhanced by the patient's involvement in the decision-making process.

Using this approach, the clinician needs to explain the treatment options to the patient so that an informed decision can be made about how to proceed. In any area of medicine, proper treatment with any medication involves four major variables, as follow.

The "Four D's"

- **Diagnosis**—Does the patient have a condition that will benefit from medication? Factors that need to be considered include:
  - Will the condition persist longer without medication?
  - Is the condition likely to progressively worsen without medication?
  - Will failure to treat with medication result in chronic residual problems or even death?
- **Drug**—The selection of the best medication is based on the safety-tolerability-efficacy-payment-simplicity (STEPS) criteria reviewed in Chapters 7 and 8.
- **Dose**—What dose will ensure the greatest likelihood of an optimal response in terms of efficacy, tolerability, and safety?
- **Duration**—An adequate trial of an antidepressant to induce a remission requires at least 4 weeks on an adequate dose. If there has not

been an adequate response by this time, then a decision to switch or augment is needed. An adequate duration for maintenance treatment is a minimum of 4 to 5 months but can be longer depending on:

– The stage of the illness
– Specific characteristics of the patient.

Some psychiatrists (this author included) recommend that if a diagnosis of major depression is made, the option of medication therapy should always be considered and offered to the patient. Nevertheless, some patients are reluctant or would prefer not to take medication if possible. Reasons include:

- The belief that taking antidepressant medication is a "sign of weakness" or "being crazy"
- Concerns about the medication itself such as:
  – Safety
  – Long-term health consequences
  – Possibility of "addiction"
- The cost of the medication.

The clinician can resolve many of these concerns through education. Currently available antidepressants are safe as established by extensive clinical trials required by the Food and Drug Administration (FDA) for registration, and by extensive clinical experience with the drugs. Antidepressants are among the most widely prescribed drugs; after only a few years on the market, the cumulative clinical experience with antidepressants often involves literally millions of patients from all walks of life under a wide range of clinical situations (eg, comorbid illnesses and treatments). Antidepressants are not addictive. The patient should not feel that s/he is "weak" or "crazy" for taking an antidepressant, but rather acknowledge that a medical condition exists that should benefit from treatment.

Nonetheless, the patient may legitimately want to know what is the evidence that the antidepressant medications will help. Those answers come from clinical trials done to gain FDA approval for marketing. In these studies, patients with major depression are randomly assigned to receive the new antidepressant, a standard antidepressant, or a placebo in a double-blind fashion (ie, neither the prescriber nor the patient knows which treatment the patient is receiving to minimize biasing the outcome). These trials typically last 6 to 8 weeks of treatment. At the end of the trial, the results are tallied to answer the following three questions:

- How many patients improved on each treatment and to what extent (ie, full remission, partial response, no response)?
- What was the incidence of adverse effects on each treatment?
  - How serious were these effects?
  - Did they persist or remit with continued treatment or require discontinuation?
- Are there any predictors of either beneficial or adverse outcome?

When evaluating results from clinical trials, the clinician should be aware that there are two common ways of reporting the results: response rates and remission rates (Table 5.1). Response rate is generally 10% to 15% higher than the remission rate. A patient who is a responder but has not experienced a full remission has benefited from treatment, but still has residual symptoms.

From such studies conducted over decades, valuable information has emerged about the treatment of major depression. There is a significant benefit to medication in terms of the likelihood of remission of the depressive episode in comparison to placebo. The number of patients who remit on placebo and on an-

52

TABLE 5.1 — WHAT IS "RESPONSE" AND "REMISSION" IN MAJOR DEPRESSION?	
Response	= 50% reduction in severity of depressive syndrome as measured by a standardized scale (eg, Hamilton Depression Rating Scale).
Remission	= A full resolution of the depressive syndrome such that the patient scores in the nondepressed range on such a standardized scale.

tidepressant therapy varies from study to study. The percentage who remit on placebo generally ranges from 20% to 30% versus a remission rate of 45% to 60% on medication. The patient's chance of responding is thus approximately doubled by taking medication.

There are features which predict placebo response (Table 5.2). The clinician can use these features when making treatment recommendations. There are also findings that do not predict placebo response.

Patients with "a reason for being depressed" do not have a higher or a poorer medication response rate

TABLE 5.2 — PREDICTORS OF PLACEBO RESPONSE IN "DEPRESSED" PATIENTS

- Mood symptom only
- Lower severity (< 15) on HDRS
- Shorter duration (< 3 months)
- Shorter interval since episode onset
- Additional psychiatric diagnoses
- Normal neuroendocrine challenge tests (eg, dexamethasone suppression test)

Abbreviations: HDRS, Hamilton Depression Rating Scale, a standardized severity assessment scale.

than do patients without "a reason." This finding, along with others, casts serious doubts on the usefulness of the concept of a "reactive depression." This term implies etiology (ie, psychosocial stress) which may be entirely spurious. The question is: Does the patient have a major depressive episode? If so, treatment is indicated.

Thus, the recommendation to use medication is based on the presence of a major depressive episode:

- The longer the episode, the more pressing the need
- The greater the severity, the more pressing the need
- The more substantial the family history, the more pressing the need.[103]

Also of importance is the fact that the decision to institute medication is just that—an empirical medication trial. If the medication produces a significant improvement within a reasonable period of time (eg, 4 weeks) and is well tolerated, then the patient and clinician will not question continuing such treatment. If the medication is not helpful, then it is appropriate to stop it and try another antidepressant as discussed in Chapter 11. Thus, the patient should understand that the decision to try medication is for a specified interval of time after which a decision can be made about whether to continue with it.

Beyond the "Four D's," patient compliance with the treatment plan is the most important factor in determining outcome of antidepressant therapy. Table 5.3 presents the variables related to noncompliance. The clinician can address and minimize many of these variables through patient education, as discussed in this section and in Chapter 4. The clinician also should determine whether other variables are present, such as:

**TABLE 5.3 — FACTORS RELATED
TO NONCOMPLIANCE**

- Duration, complexity, and tolerability of regimen
- Lack of trust
- Lack of supportive follow-up
- Perceived mastery over the illness
- Severity of the illness
- Doubts about effectiveness
- Lack of social supports
- Poor educational background
- Organicity
- Concomitant substance abuse

- The occurrence of rate-limiting adverse effects
- Lack of social support
- The concomitant presence of substance abuse and/or organicity.

If these variables are present, the clinician needs to address them and modify the treatment plan accordingly.

In terms of education, the patient should understand that without effective treatment, the episode may last for many months to even several years. Such a prolonged episode can cause considerable functional impairment, both in the patient's personal life and on the job.

The patient should also understand what is expected from treatment. The goal is full remission of the depressive episode on monodrug therapy. This goal is realistic for a substantial percentage of patients in the primary-care setting.

6

The Rational Basis for the Development and Use of Newer Antidepressants

A decade ago, the practitioner had limited options for treating patients with clinical depression. Those options were:

- Tricyclic antidepressants (TCAs)
- Monoamine oxidase inhibitors (MAOIs)
- Trazodone. *(Desyrel)*

The practitioner now has 22 different antidepressants from eight different mechanistically defined classes of antidepressants (Table 6.1).

This chapter will explain how this mechanistically based classification system can be used to conceptualize the clinical relevance of the various antidepressants available to treat patients. Thus, this chapter can be used as a reference when reading subsequent chapters. The goal is to summarize the knowledge necessary to:

- Predict the clinical effects of different antidepressants
- Choose a specific antidepressant for a specific patient based on those predicted effects
- Rationally think about sequential treatment options for the patient who has not benefited from a trial of a specific type of antidepressant
- Anticipate potential drug-drug interactions when using a specific antidepressant in combination with other medications.

**.1 — CLASSIFICATION OF
JEPRESSANTS BY PUTATIVE
NISM(S) OF ACTION RESPONSIBLE
R ANTIDEPRESSANT EFFICACY:***
ERIC/(TRADE) NAMES BY DRUG CLASS

Mixed Reuptake and Neuroreceptor Antagonists[†]

- Amitriptyline (Elavil)
- Amoxapine (Ascendin)
- Clomipramine (Anafranil)
- Doxepin (Sinequan)
- Imipramine (Tofranil-PM)
- Trimipramine (Surmontil)

Norepinephrine Selective Reuptake Inhibitors (NSRIs)[‡]
- Desipramine (Norpramin) TCA
- Maprotiline (Ludiomil)
- Nortriptyline (Pamelor, Aventyl)
- Protriptyline (Vivactil)

Serotonin Selective Reuptake Inhibitors (SSRIs)
- Citalopram (Celexa)
- Fluoxetine (Prozac)
- Fluvoxamine (Luvox)
- Paroxetine (Paxil)
- Sertraline (Zoloft)

*Serotonin and Norepinephrine
Reuptake Inhibitor (SNRI)*[§]
- Venlafaxine (Effexor)

*Serotonin-2A (5-HT2A) Receptor Blocker
and Weak Serotonin Uptake Inhibitor*[∥]
- Nefazodone (Serzone)
- Trazodone (Desyrel)

*Serotonin (5-HT2A and 2C) and
α_{-2} Norepinephrine Receptor Blocker*[∥]
- Mirtazapine (Remeron)

Dopamine and Norepinephrine Reuptake Inhibitors
- Bupropion (Wellbutrin, Wellbutrin SR, Zyban Sustained-Release)

Monoamine Oxidase Inhibitors (MAOIs)[¶]
- Phenelzine (Nardil)
- Tranylcypromine (Parnate)

Abbreviations: 5-HT, 5-hydroxytryptamine (serotonin).

* The presumptive mechanism of action for each drug is based on the preclinical pharmacology of the drug and the fact that it and/or its active metabolites reach sufficient concentration *in vivo* to affect this site of action, given its *in vitro* potency.

† All of these drugs are tertiary amine tricyclic antidepressants (TCAs) except amoxapine.

‡ All of these drugs are secondary amine TCAs except maprotiline. There are nontricyclic NSRIs available in other parts of the world, such as reboxetine. Those drugs share the ability to inhibit norepinephrine uptake with the secondary amine TCAs and maprotiline but do not carry the risk of serious toxicity even after a substantial overdose.

§ At present, venlafaxine is the only member of this class available in the United States although several others are in various stages of clinical testing.

‖ Both nefazodone and mirtazapine also have other mechanisms of action that are engaged at concentrations which occur under clinically relevant dosing guidelines (see Table 6.2).

¶ Only irreversible and nonselective monoamine oxidase inhibitors (MAOIs) are available in the United States, but selective and reversible MAOIs are marketed elsewhere in the world.

Rational Drug Development

Drug development in psychiatry has evolved from a process based on chance to one based on molecularly targeting specific sites of action in the central nervous system (CNS) (ie, specific neuroreceptors or neuronal uptake pumps for neurotransmitters). The goal of such development is to affect only mechanisms mediating antidepressant efficacy while simultaneously avoiding affects on other mechanisms which mediate tolerability and/or safety problems.[181,183,236] The intent is to produce antidepressants which are:

- Safer
- Better tolerated
- Less likely to interact with other coprescribed drugs than was the case with the older agents (ie, TCAs, MAOIs and trazodone).

The success of this approach is underscored by the fact that the risk of the clinical depression is now clearly worse than the risk of the treatment such that even a hint of clinical depression may be sufficient to warrant an empirical trial of a newer antidepressant. That explains the substantial expansion in the use of antidepressants that has occurred over the last decade.[164]

The eight functional pharmacologic classes of antidepressants based on their presumed mechanism(s) of antidepressant action are listed in Table 6.1. Table 6.2 indicates which mechanisms of action are engaged by these different antidepressants at their usually effective antidepressant dose. In Table 6.3, the clinical consequences that occur as a result of blocking specific sites of action are listed. By using Tables 6.2 and 6.3 in combination, the clinician can determine what specific effects a particular antidepressant will produce in the usual patient on the usual antidepressant dose. Tables 6.4 through 6.7 summarize the usual adverse effects produced by these various drugs based on the results of double-blind, placebo-controlled clinical trials. These tables will serve as reference points throughout the remainder of the book.

Relationship Between Pharmacodynamics, Pharmacokinetics and Interindividual Variability

The nature and magnitude of a drug's effect is determined by its:

- Site of action
- Binding affinity for that site
- Concentration at the site.[170]

These factors determine the "usual" effect of the drug in the "usual" patient on the "usual" dose as determined in a clinical trial. However, all patients are not "usual" due to interindividual variability caused by factors such as:

- Age
- Genetics
- Gender
- Intercurrent diseases affecting organ function
- Concomitant drug therapy
- Social habits (eg, smoking).[131]

The clinician must take into account how a specific patient may differ from the "usual" patient in a clinical trial when selecting and dosing a drug. The three important variables determining the effect of a drug on a patient are summarized in the following equation:

(Equation 1)

Effect =
pharmacodynamics × pharmacokinetics × interindividual variance

This equation can be restated as follows:

(Equation 2)

Effect =
potency for × concentration at × interindividual
site of action   site of action   variance

TABLE 6.2 — COMPARISON OF THE MECHANISMS OF ACTION OF ANTIDEPRESSANTS*

Mechanism of Action[†]	Amitriptyline	Desipramine	Sertraline	Venlafaxine	Nefazodone	Mirtazapine	Bupropion	Tranylcypromine
Histamine-1 receptor blockade	Yes[‡]	No	No	No	No	Yes[‡]	No	No
Acetylcholine receptor blockade	Yes	No	No	No	No	No	No	No
NE uptake inhibition	Yes	Yes	No	Yes	No	No	Yes	No
5-HT2A receptor blockade	Yes	No	No	No	Yes[‡]	Yes	No	No
α_{-1} NE receptor blockade	Yes	No	No	No	Yes	No	No	No
5-HT uptake inhibition	Yes	No	Yes	Yes[‡]	Yes	No	No	No
α_{-2} NE receptor blockade	No	No	No	Yes[‡]	No	Yes	No	No
5-HT2C receptor blockade	No	No	No	No	No	Yes	No	No
5-HT3 receptor blockade	No	No	No	No	No	Yes	No	No
Fast Na$^+$ channels inhibition	No	No	No	No	No	No	No	No

Dopamine uptake inhibition	No	No	No	No	No	Yes	No
Monoamine oxidase inhibition	No	No	No	No	No	No	Yes

Abbreviations: NE, norepinephrine; 5-HT, 5-hydroxytryptamine (serotonin); Na⁺, sodium.

* Amitriptyline represents the mixed reuptake and neuroreceptor blocking class, desipramine—norepinephrine selective reuptake inhibitors, sertraline—serotonin selective reuptake inhibitors, venlafaxine—serotonin and norepinephrine reuptake inhibitors, nefazodone—5-HT2A and weak serotonin uptake inhibitors and mirtazapine—specific serotonin and norepinephrine receptor blockers, bupropion—dopamine and norepinephrine uptake inhibitor. Monoamine oxidase inhibitors (MAOIs) do not directly share any mechanism of action with other classes of antidepressants, although they affect dopamine, norepinephrine, and serotonin neurotransmission via their effects on monoamine oxidase.

† The effects of these various antidepressants are listed using a binary (yes/no) approach for simplicity and clinical relevance. The issue for clinician and patient is whether the effect is expected under usual dosing conditions. A "yes" means that the usual patient on the usually effective antidepressant dose of the drug achieves concentrations of parent drug and/or metabolites that should engage that specific target to a physiologically/clinically significant extent given the *in vitro* affinity of the parent drug and/or metabolites for that target. If the affinity for another target is within an order of magnitude of desired target, then that target is likely also affected to a physiologically relevant degree. For example, under usual dosing conditions, amitriptyline achieves concentrations that engage the norepinephrine uptake pump. At such concentrations, it also substantially blocks histamine-1 and muscarinic acetylcholine

Continued

receptors since it has even more affinity for those targets than it does for the norepinephrine uptake pump. Since the binding affinity of amitriptyline for the 5-HT2A and α_{-1} norepinephrine receptors and the serotonin uptake pump are within an order of magnitude of its affinity for the norepinephrine uptake pump, amitriptyline at usual therapeutic concentrations for antidepressant efficacy will also affect those targets. On the other hand, amitriptyline will not typically affect Na$^+$ fast channels at usual therapeutic concentrations because there is more than an order of magnitude (ie, > ten-fold) separation between its effects on this target versus norepinephrine uptake inhibition. Nevertheless, an amitriptyline overdose can result in concentrations which engage this target. That fact accounts for the narrow therapeutic index of the tricyclic antidepressants (TCAs) and is the reason therapeutic drug monitoring to detect unusually slow clearance is a standard of care when using such drugs.

‡ Most potent effect (ie, effect that occurs at lowest concentration). See previous footnote for further explanation.

The binding affinities of all drugs listed in the table (except mirtazapine) are based on the work of Cusack et al and Bolden-Watson and Richelson. Information on the binding affinities of mirtazapine (including affinities for 5-HT2A and 5-HT3 receptors) is based on the work of de Boer et al. Although the publications by the Richelson group did not include values for the 5-HT2A and 5-HT3 receptors or the other antidepressants, Elliot Richelson of the Mayo Clinic in Jacksonville, Florida (personal communication) confirmed that the other antidepressants would be unlikely to affect these receptors under usual dosing conditions.

Adapted from: Bolden-Watson C, Richelson E. *Life Sci.* 1993;52:1023-1029; Cusack B, et al. *Psychopharmacology.* 1994;114:559-565; de Boer T, et al. *Neuropharmacology.* 1988;27:399-408; de Boer T, et al. *Hum Psychopharmacol.* 1995;10:107S-118S; and Frazer A. *J Clin Psychiatry.* 1997;58(suppl 6):9-25.

The first two terms in this equation explain the relationship between pharmacodynamics and pharmacokinetics. The first term determines the nature of the drug's effect and how much drug is needed at the site of action to engage that site to a clinically meaningful extent in the usual patient. The second term in the equation determines the magnitude of the drug's effect by determining how much drug reaches the site of action. The third term explains how interindividual variability in the patient can shift the dose-response curve (ie, greater or lesser effect than usually expected relative to the dose prescribed).

The following equation explains how dose is related to the drug concentration, which is the second term in Equation 2:

(Equation 3)

Concentration = dosing rate (mg/day)/clearance (mL/min)

In other words, the concentration achieved in a specific patient is determined by the dosage of the drug the patient is taking relative to the patient's ability to clear the drug from the body.

Pharmacodynamic Principles Central to Understanding Antidepressant Options

As a general rule, most drugs (including antidepressants) act as antagonists at their site(s) of action. Table 6.3 shows the effects produced by blocking a specific neural mechanism. If a drug were to act as an agonist at a specific site, then it would produce the opposite effect to that shown in Table 6.3.

Antidepressants which block neuronal uptake pumps for serotonin, norepinephrine and dopamine act as indirect agonists by increasing the concentration of these neurotransmitters at their respective receptors. Thus, the clinical effects of uptake inhibitors will be

TABLE 6.3 — SITES OF ACTION AND CLINICAL AND PHYSIOLOGIC CONSEQUENCES OF BLOCKADE OR ANTAGONISM

Site of Action	Consequence of Blockade
Histamine-1 receptor	Sedation, antipruritic effect
Muscarinic acetylcholine receptor	Dry mouth, constipation, sinus tachycardia, memory impairment
NE uptake pump	Antidepressant efficacy, ↑ blood pressure, tremors, diaphoresis
5-HT2A receptor	Antidepressant efficacy, ↑ rapid eye movement sleep, antianxiety efficacy, anti-extrapyramidal symptoms
α-$_1$ NE receptor	Orthostatic hypotension, sedation
5-HT2 uptake pump	Antidepressant efficacy, nausea, loose stools, insomnia, anorgasmia
α-$_2$ NE receptor	Antidepressant efficacy, arousal, ↑ libido
5-HT2C receptor	Antianxiety efficacy, ↑ appetite, ↓ motor restlessness
5-HT3 receptor	Antinauseant
Fast Na$^+$ channels	Delayed repolarization leading to arrhythmia, seizures, delirium

Dopamine uptake pump	Antidepressant efficacy, euphoria, abuse potential, antiparkinson activity, aggravation of psychosis
Monoamine oxidase	Antidepressant activity, decreased blood pressure*

Abbreviations: NE, norepinephrine; 5-HT, 5-hydroxytryptamine (serotonin); Na⁺, sodium.

* Hypertensive crisis (ie, markedly elevated blood pressure) and serotonin syndrome can occur when monoamine oxidase inhibitors are combined with noradrenergic and serotonin agonists, respectively.

Adapted from: Preskorn SH. *Clinical Pharmacology of Selective Serotonin Reuptake Inhibitors.* Caddo, Okla: Professional Communications, Inc; 1996:48-49.

TABLE 6.4 — COMPARISON OF THE PLACEBO-SUBTRACTED INCIDENCE RATE (%) OF FREQUENT ADVERSE EFFECTS FOR CITALOPRAM, FLUOXETINE, FLUVOXAMINE, PAROXETINE, AND SERTRALINE*[†]

Adverse Effect	Citalopram (n=1063, n=446)[a]	Fluoxetine (n=1730, n=799)[a]	Fluvoxamine (n=222, n=192)[a]	Paroxetine (n=421, n=421)[a]	Sertraline (n=861, n=853)[a]
Anorexia	2	7.2	8.6	4.5	1.2
Confusion[b]	NA	1.5	NA	1	0.8
Constipation	< placebo	1.2	11.2	5.2	2.1
Diarrhea[c]	3	5.3	− 0.4	4	8.4
Dizziness[d]	< placebo	4	1.3	7.8	5
Drowsiness[e]	8	5.9	17.2	14.3	7.5
Dry mouth	6	3.5	1.8	6	7
Dyspepsia	1	2.1	3.2	0.9	3.2
Fatigue[f]	2	5.6	6.2	10.3	2.5

Flatulence	NA	0.5	NA	2.3	0.8
Frequent micturition	NA	1.6	0.6	2.4	0.8
Headache	< placebo	4.8	2.9	0.3	1.3
Increased appetite	NA	NA	NA	NA	NA
Insomnia	1	6.7	4	7.1	7.6
Nausea[g]	8	11	25.6	16.4	14.3
Nervousness[h]	3	10.3	7.6	4.9	4.4
Palpitations[i]	< placebo	−0.1	NA	1.5	1.9
Paresthesia[j]	NA	−0.3	NA	2.1	1.3
Rash[k]	NA	0.9	NA	1	0.6
Respiratory[l]	8	5.8	−1.3	0.8	0.8
Sweating	2	4.6	−1.3	8.8	5.5

Continued

6

Adverse Effect	Citalopram ($n=1063$, $n=446$)[a]	Fluoxetine ($n=1730$, $n=799$)[a]	Fluvoxamine ($n=222$, $n=192$)[a]	Paroxetine ($n=421$, $n=421$)[a]	Sertraline ($n=861$, $n=853$)[a]
Tremors	2	5.5	6.1	6.4	8
Urinary retention[m]	< placebo	NA	NA	2.7	0.9
Vision disturbances	< placebo	1	0	2.2	2.1
Weight gain	NA	NA	NA	NA	NA

Abbreviations: NA, not available.

* Data for fluoxetine, paroxetine and sertraline is from Preskorn SH. *J Clin Psychiatry*. 1995;56(suppl 6):12-21; data for fluvoxamine is from *Compendium of Pharmaceuticals and Specialties*. 33rd ed. 1998:922-924; data for citalopram is from Forest Pharmaceuticals, Inc. prescribing information; 1998. Incidence of each respective adverse effect for patients taking each drug minus the incidence for each drug's parallel placebo control in double-blind, placebo-controlled studies.

† The above adverse effect data come from product labeling as opposed to head-to-head trials. Such data may not necessarily reflect the actual rate of these adverse effects in clinical practice or the actual differences between these various drugs.

a The first value is the number of patients on that medication, while the second represents those treated in the parallel, placebo group.

b Includes decreased concentration, memory impairment, abandoned thinking concentration.

c Includes gastroenteritis.

d Includes lightheadedness, postural hypotension, and hypotension.

e Includes somnolence, sedation, and drugged feeling.

f Includes asthenia, myasthenia, and psychomotor retardation.

g Includes vomiting.

h Includes anxiety, agitation, hostility, akathisia, and central nervous system stimulation.

i Includes tachycardia and arrhythmias.

j Includes sensation disturbances and hypesthesia.

k Includes pruritus.

l Includes respiratory disorder, upper respiratory infection, flu, dyspnea, pharyngitis, sinus congestion, oropharynx disorder, fever, and chill.

m Includes micturition disorder, difficulty with micturition, and urinary hesitancy.

TABLE 6.5 — COMPARISON OF THE PLACEBO-SUBTRACTED INCIDENCE RATE (%) OF FREQUENT ADVERSE EFFECTS FOR BUPROPION, IMIPRAMINE, MIRTAZAPINE, NEFAZODONE, AND VENLAFAXINE[*][†]

Adverse Effect	Bupropion (n=323, n=185)[a]	Imipramine (n=367, n=672)[a]	Mirtazapine (n=453, n=361)[a]	Nefazodone (n=393, n=394)[a]	Venlafaxine-IR (n=1033, n=609)[a]	Venlafaxine-XR (n=357, n=285)[a]
Anorexia	− 0.1	NA	NA	NA	9	4
Confusion[b]	2.8	NA	2	9	1	2
Constipation	8.7	17.4	6	6	8	3
Diarrhea[c]	− 1.8	− 2.7	< placebo	1	1	< placebo
Dizziness[d]	6.8	22.7	4	23	12	11
Drowsiness[e]	0.3	12	36	11	14	9
Dry mouth	9.2	47.1	10	12	11	6
Dyspepsia	0.9	NA	< placebo	2	1	< placebo

Fatigue[f]	− 3.6	7.6	3	7	6	1
Flatulence	NA	NA	< placebo	NA	1	1
Frequent micturition	0.3	NA	1	1	1	NA
Headache	3.5	− 8.7	< placebo	3	1	< placebo
Increased appetite	NA	NA	15	NA	1	2
Insomnia	5.3	0.4	< placebo	2	8	6
Nausea[g]	4	1.3	< placebo	11	26	21
Nervousness[h]	13.9	3.6	< placebo	NA	12	7
Palpitations[i]	4.7	NA	< placebo	NA	2	< placebo
Paresthesia[j]	0.8	NA	NA	2	1	NA
Rash[k]	3.7	NA	NA	2	1	NA
Respiratory[l]	− 2.5	− 2.3	3	9	NA	1

Continued

Adverse Effect	Bupropion (n=323, n=185)[a]	Imipramine (n=367, n=672)[a]	Mirtazapine (n=453, n=361)[a]	Nefazodone (n=393, n=394)[a]	Venlafaxine-IR (n=1033, n=609)[a]	Venlafaxine-XR (n = 357, n = 285)[a]
Sweating	7.7	11.2	< placebo	NA	9	11
Tremors	13.5	10	1	1	4	3
Urinary retention[m]	− 0.3	4	NA	1	2	NA
Vision disturbances	4.3	5.4	< placebo	12	4	4
Weight gain	NA	NA	10	NA	NA	NA

Abbreviations: IR, immediate release; XR, extended release; NA, not available.

* Data from Preskorn SH. *J Clin Psychiatry*. 1995;56(suppl 6):12-21; Remeron (mirtazapine). *Physicians' Desk Reference*; 1999:2147-2149; and Effexor (venlafaxine hydrochloride). *Physicians' Desk Reference*; 1999:3298-3302.

† The above adverse effect data come from product labeling as opposed to head-to-head trials. Such data may not necessarily reflect the actual rate of these adverse effects in clinical practice or the actual differences between these various drugs.

a The first value is the number of patients on that medication, while the second represents those treated in the parallel, placebo group.

b Includes decreased concentration, memory impairment, and abandoned thinking concentration.

c Includes gastroenteritis.

d Includes lightheadedness, postural hypotension, and hypotension.

e Includes somnolence, sedation, and drugged feeling.

f Includes asthenia, myasthenia, and psychomotor retardation.

g Includes vomiting.

h Includes anxiety, agitation, hostility, akathisia, and central nervous system stimulation.

i Includes tachycardia and arrhythmias.

j Includes sensation disturbances and hypesthesia.

k Includes pruritus.

l Includes respiratory disorder, upper respiratory infection, flu, dyspnea, pharyngitis, sinus congestion, oropharynx disorder, fever, and chill.

m Includes micturition disorder, difficulty with micturition, and urinary hesitancy.

TABLE 6.6 — THE MOST LIKELY SPECIFIC ADVERSE EFFECTS ON SPECIFIC SSRIS ABOVE AND BEYOND THE PARALLEL PLACEBO CONDITION
(PERCENTAGE ON DRUG MINUS PERCENTAGE ON PLACEBO BASED ON REGISTRATION STUDIES)*†‡

SSRI	>7.5%	>10%	>15%	>20%	>25%	>30%	>35%	>40%	>45%
Citalopram	Drowsiness Respiratory Nausea	—	—	—	—	—	—	—	—
Fluoxetine	—	Nausea Nervousness	—	—	—	—	—	—	—
Fluvoxamine	Anorexia	Constipation	Drowsiness	—	Nausea	—	—	—	—
Paroxetine	Dizziness Sweating	Fatigue	Drowsiness Nausea	—	—	—	—	—	—
Sertraline	Insomnia Diarrhea	Nausea	—	—	—	—	—	—	—

Abbreviations: SSRI, serotonin selective reuptake inhibitors.

* Best available data also suggests that all SSRIs can cause sexual dysfunction (eg. delayed ejaculation, decreased libido, anorgasmia) in approximately 30% of patients.

† This table is based on Table 6.4.

‡ The above adverse effect data come from product labeling as opposed to head-to-head trials. Such data may not necessarily reflect the actual rate of these adverse effects in clinical practice or the actual differences between these various drugs.

the opposite of those shown in Table 6.3. For example, by increasing the availability of serotonin or 5-hydroxytryptamine (5-HT) receptors, serotonin reuptake inhibitors (SRIs) act as indirect agonists at the following receptors:

- 5-HT2A
- 5-HT2C
- 5-HT3.[83]

As outlined in Table 6.2, SRIs include all of the serotonin selective reuptake inhibitors (SSRIs) and the serotonin and norepinephrine reuptake inhibitor (SNRI), venlafaxine. (*Effexor*)

The above helps to explain why all SRIs can:

- Decrease rapid eye movement (REM) sleep and shift sleep architecture from restorative, deep stage IV sleep to light stage I sleep due to indirect stimulation of the 5-HT2A receptor[9,159,217,226,230]
- Decrease appetite and cause motor restlessness due to indirect stimulation of the 5-HT2C receptor[238]
- Cause nausea by indirect stimulation of the 5-HT3 receptor.[83]

The indirect stimulation of one of these 5-HT receptors (or perhaps another) likely mediates the sexual dysfunction seen with all SSRIs, including:

- Anorgasmia
- Delayed ejaculation
- Decrease libido.[145,147]

The reverse logic explains the effects of other antidepressants. For example, nefazodone (*Serzone*) and mirtazapine (*Remeron*) can increase stage IV sleep most likely by blocking the 5-HT2A receptor.[214] Mirtazapine can also increase appetite and decrease motor restlessness by blocking the 5-HT2C receptor and can treat nausea

Antidepressant	>7.5%	>10%	>15%	>20%	>25%	>30%	>35%	>40%	>45%
Bupropion (Wellbutrin)	Dry mouth Constipation Sweating	—	—	—	—	—	—	—	—
Imipramine (Tofranil)	Fatigue	Tremors Sweating	Constipation	Dizziness	—	—	—	—	Dry mouth
Mirtazapine (Remeron)	—	Weight gain Dry mouth	↑ Appetite	—	—	—	Drowsiness	—	—
Nefazodone (Serzone)	Confusion Respiratory	Drowsiness Vision disturbance Nausea Dry mouth	—	Dizziness	—	—	—	—	—

TABLE 6.7 — THE MOST LIKELY SPECIFIC ADVERSE EFFECTS ON SPECIFIC ANTIDEPRESSANTS ABOVE AND BEYOND THE PARALLEL PLACEBO CONDITION (PERCENTAGE ON DRUG MINUS PERCENTAGE ON PLACEBO BASED ON REGISTRATION STUDIES)*†

NRI

SNRB

Venlafaxine-IR (Effexor)	Insomnia Anorexia Constipation Sweating	Nervousness Dizziness Dry mouth	Drowsiness	—	Nausea	—	—	—
Venlafaxine-XR (Effexor)	Nervousness Drowsiness	Sweating Dizziness	—	Nausea	—	—	—	—

Abbreviations: IR, immediate release; XR, extended release.

* This table is based on Table 6.5.

† The above adverse effect data come from product labeling as opposed to head-to-head trials. Such data may not necessarily reflect the actual rate of these adverse effects in clinical practice or the actual differences between these various drugs.

SNRI

by blocking the 5-HT3 receptor.[83] Trazodone is also a 5-HT2A blocker which is consistent with its widespread use as an antidote for the sleep disturbances that occur in some patients on SRIs.[155] In addition, the effects of mirtazapine and trazodone on sleep are further amplified by their shared ability to block central histamine receptors.[31,54,58,59,77] The fact that nefazodone and mirtazapine cause minimal, if any, sexual dysfunction is consistent with their minimal inhibition of serotonin uptake perhaps coupled with their blockade of the 5-HT2A receptor.[31,54,58,59,77] These issues are further discussed in Chapters 8 and 11.

Some antidepressants, like SSRIs, directly affect only one site of action at the usual concentration achieved under therapeutic dosing conditions; other antidepressants affect more than one site. As shown in Table 6.1, venlafaxine and nefazodone affect more than one site; the same is also true for bupropion. Tertiary amine tricyclic antidepressants (TATCAs), such as amitriptyline, affect six different targets at usual therapeutic concentrations.

Drugs which affect more than one site of action often act sequentially (ie, as their concentration increases, they affect additional targets) which explains why these drugs exhibit different effects to different degrees at different doses. Figure 6.1 illustrates this pharmacologic principle: amitriptyline can affect multiple sites of action, in contrast to desipramine and sertraline which are selective for a single (although different) neural site of action. Parenthetically, some SSRIs (eg, fluoxetine) affect cytochrome P450 (CYP) enzymes, which are non-neural sites of action with important pharmacokinetic drug-drug interaction consequences (Figure 6.2). This issue is discussed in greater detail in Chapters 8 and 10.

The multiple actions of the TATCAs (eg, amitriptyline, doxepin, imipramine, trimipramine), like the effects of some newer antidepressants on CYP en-

80

FIGURE 6.1 — RELATIVE POTENCY FOR DIFFERENT SITES OF ACTION FOR THREE DIFFERENT TYPES OF ANTIDEPRESSANTS: AMITRIPTYLINE, DESIPRAMINE, AND SERTRALINE

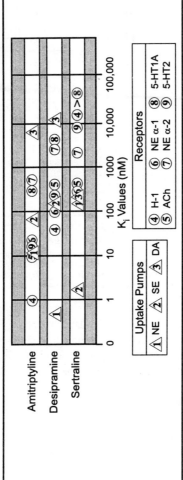

Abbreviations: NE, norepinephrine; SE, serotonin; DA, dopamine; H-1, histamine; ACh, acetylcholine; 5-HT, 5-hydroxy-tryptamine (serotonin).

Based on data from: Bolden-Watson C, Richelson E. *Life Sci.* 1993;52:1023-1029 and Cusack B, et al. *Psychopharmacology.* 1994;114:559-565.

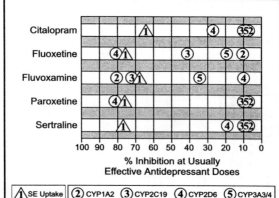

FIGURE 6.2 — *IN VIVO* **PROFILE
OF SSRIs ON SE UPTAKE INHIBITION
VERSUS CYP ENZYME INHIBITION**

% Inhibition at Usually
Effective Antidepressant Doses

⚠ SE Uptake   ② CYP1A2   ③ CYP2C19   ④ CYP2D6   ⑤ CYP3A3/4

Abbreviations: SSRI, serotonin selective reuptake inhibitor; SE, serotonin; CYP, cytochrome P450 enzyme.

Based on data from: Shad MU, Preskorn SH. In: Levy R, et al, eds. Philadelphia, Pa: Lippincott, Williams &Wilkins. In press.

zymes, are now generally considered to be a clinical disadvantage.[170,171] To understand the pharmacology of amitriptyline, imagine the number of single mechanism of action drugs the patient would have to take to achieve all the effects that can be obtained with amitriptyline alone (Table 6.8). At low doses (or concentrations), amitriptyline blocks histamine receptors; at higher doses, amitriptyline sequentially blocks the other sites as illustrated in Figure 6.1 and enumerated in Tables 6.2 and 6.3.

The pharmacology of TATCAs such as amitriptyline served as the blueprint for what effects newer antidepressants should and should not have and, thus, amitriptyline also served as the basis for the classifi-

TABLE 6.8 — AMITRIPTYLINE: POLYDRUG THERAPY IN A SINGLE PILL

Drug	Action
Chlorpheniramine	Histamine-1 receptor blockade
Cimetidine	Histamine-2 receptor blockade
Benztropine	Acetylcholine receptor blockade
Desipramine	NE uptake inhibition
Nefazodone	5-HT2A receptor blockade
Sertraline	Serotonin uptake inhibition
Prazosin	α_1 NE receptor blockade
Yohimbine	α_2 NE receptor blockade
Quinidine	Direct membrane stabilization

Abbreviations: NE, norepinephrine; 5-HT, 5-hydroxy-tryptamine (serotonin).

cation system presented in Table 6.1.[181,236] Table 6.2 lists specific neural mechanisms in the order in which they are affected by amitriptyline; the most potent mechanism (histamine receptor blockade) being listed at the top and the least potent (inhibition of sodium [Na^+] fast channels) listed near the bottom. The latter action occurs at drug concentrations approximately 10 times higher than those needed to block neural uptake pumps for norepinephrine and serotonin. While inhibition of neural uptake pumps for these chemical transmitters is believed to be responsible for the antidepressant efficacy of the TATCAs, the inhibition of Na^+ fast channels results in slowing of intracardiac conduction and hence can cause fatal arrhythmias. The potency of TATCAs for this site of action explains why only modest overdoses can be lethal in suicide attempts.[194]

One goal of rational drug development with regard to newer antidepressants was to widen the therapeutic index by avoiding the inhibition of Na^+ fast channels.[170] Another goal was to avoid the adverse effects of TATCAs, which can be troublesome even if not seriously toxic. For example, all of the SSRIs share with TATCAs the ability to block the neural uptake of serotonin, but do not share the ability to block histamine, muscarinic cholinergic and alpha-1–adrenergic receptors. For this reason, SSRIs avoid the adverse effects of sedation, constipation and orthostatic hypotension which plague the users of TATCAs (Figure 6.3). Other newer antidepressants engage other neural targets at concentrations achieved under clinically relevant dosing conditions (Figure 6.4 and Table 6.2).

Pharmacodynamic Drug-Drug Interactions

The clinician can also use Tables 6.2 and 6.3 to anticipate what type of pharmacodynamically mediated drug interactions are likely to occur when a specific type of antidepressant is used in combination with other agents. For example, all SSRIs can interact with MAOIs to cause the serotonin syndrome.[51,87,144,158,228,233] Similarly, all antidepressants that centrally block the histamine receptor potentiate the adverse cognitive-motor effects of alcohol.[140,151,192] All antidepressants that block the alpha-1–adrenergic receptor have the potential to aggravate the orthostatic hypotension caused by other antihypertensive medications.[103,192]

Serotonin syndrome!

FIGURE 6.3 — RELATIVE POTENCY FOR DIFFERENT SITES OF ACTION FOR THE VARIOUS MEMBERS OF THE SSRI CLASS OF ANTIDEPRESSANTS

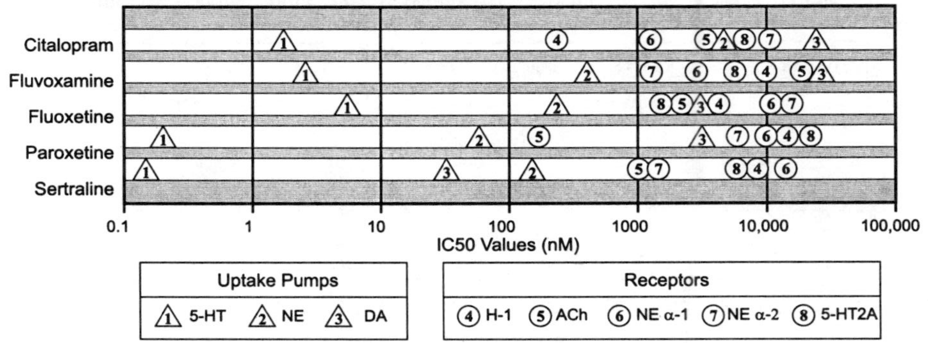

Abbreviations: SSRI, serotonin selective reuptake inhibitor; 5-HT, 5-hydroxytryptamine (serotonin); NE, norepinephrine; DA, dopamine; H-1, histamine; ACh, acetylcholine.

Based on data from: Hyttel J. *Nord J Psychiatry*. 1993;47(suppl 30)5-12.

FIGURE 6.4 — RELATIVE POTENCY FOR DIFFERENT SITES OF ACTION FOR NON-SSRI ANTIDEPRESSANTS: BUPROPION, IMIPRAMINE, MIRTAZAPINE, NEFAZODONE, AND VENLAFAXINE

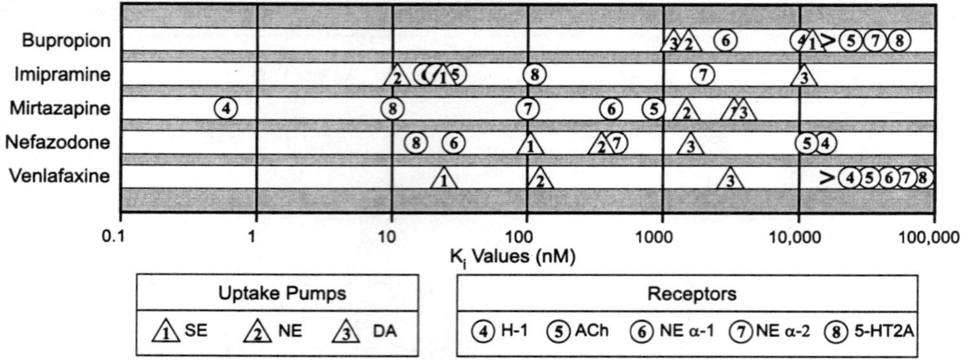

Abbreviations: SE, serotonin; NE, norepinephrine; DA, dopamine; H-1, histamine; ACh, acetylcholine; 5-HT, 5-hydroxytryptamine (serotonin).

Based on data from: Bolden-Watson C, Richelson E. *Life Sci.* 1993;52:1023-1029; Cusack B, et al. *Psychopharmacology.* 1994;114:559-565; de Boer T, et al. *Neuropharmacology.* 1988;27:399-408; and de Boer T, et al. *Hum Psychopharmacol.* 1995;10:107S-118S.

A Non-neural Target: Cytochrome P450 Enzymes

As mentioned earlier, CYP enzymes can be a site of action for a drug.[93,94] Although CYP enzymes may be unintended and unnecessary targets for an antidepressant, they are clinically important because inhibition of these enzymes (Figure 6.2) carries with it the liability for causing specific types of pharmacokinetic drug-drug interactions.

While newer antidepressants were designed to selectively affect specific neural targets (eg, a specific intake pump) and avoid others (eg, muscarinic cholinergic receptors), they were not rationally designed to avoid the inhibition of CYP enzymes. The reason is simple: the newer antidepressants were developed before the isolation of the first CYP enzyme in 1988.[84] In fact, the newer antidepressants were synthesized and screened against targets known in the mid- to late 1970s. Since it is not possible to avoid "hitting" what is not known, some of the new antidepressants have subsequently been found to unintentionally inhibit one or more drug-metabolizing CYP enzyme to a clinically meaningful degree (Figure 6.2 and Table 6.6).

The five major CYP enzymes mediating oxidative drug metabolism (in order of importance) are:

- CYP 3A3/4 *50 %*
- CYP 2D6 *30 %*
- CYP 1A2
- CYP 2C9/10
- CYP 2C19.[93,94,223]

Of these, CYP 3A3/4 and CYP 2D6 are responsible for approximately 50% and 30% of known oxidative drug metabolism, respectively.[115,255]

Since the isolation of the first CYP enzyme, knowledge in this area has exploded. Drugs such as terfenadine (Seldane) and mibefradil (Posicor) have been withdrawn from the US market as a result of CYP enzyme-mediated drug interactions. Testing for effects on CYP enzymes is now part of rational drug development and is done to avoid developing new agents that inadvertently inhibit these enzymes.[170] Similar testing is also being done on currently available drugs to determine which CYP enzymes are important for their clearance and whether they induce or inhibit specific CYP enzymes.

Such testing is generally done in two steps:

- First, an *in vitro* approach is used to determine the ability of a CYP enzyme to metabolize a drug (Table 6.9) and conversely to estimate the potential (ie, potency) for a new candidate drug to inhibit a CYP enzyme
- Second, formal drug-drug interaction studies in humans are performed to establish whether clinically meaningful inhibition occurs under usual dosing conditions (Tables 6.10 and 6.11).[93,94,223]

This technology thus yields two sets of complementary data that can be used to predict clinically meaningful CYP enzyme-mediated drug interactions, as illustrated in Figure 6.5:

- The first set of data determine whether a drug inhibits a specific CYP enzyme and to what extent under clinically relevant dosing conditions.
- The second set of data establish which drugs are dependent on which CYP enzyme for oxidative metabolism.

Table 6.10 summarizes the effects of newer antidepressants on these five CYP enzymes. Table 6.9 lists the drugs known to be metabolized by these CYP enzymes.

The principal distinguishing characteristic among the various SSRIs is their differential effects on CYP enzymes.[93,94,170,223] While all five drugs block the neural uptake of serotonin and avoid effects on other neural targets, they differ substantially with regard to their effects on CYP enzymes. Fluoxetine, fluvoxamine and paroxetine all inhibit one or more CYP enzymes to a clinically significant degree at their usually effective antidepressant dose, whereas citalopram and sertraline do not. Since the inhibition of CYP enzymes conveys no clinical benefit to the best of our knowledge, the absence of substantial effects on CYP enzymes conveys a distinct advantage for citalopram and sertraline relative to other SSRIs.

6

Pharmacodynamic Principles Central to Understanding Antidepressant Options

In general, all antidepressants are similar with regard to a number of pharmacokinetic parameters (ie, absorption and distribution). The clinically important pharmacokinetic differences among these drugs include:

- Which CYP enzymes mediate their metabolism? This information is listed in Table 6.9 and can be used to predict CYP enzyme-mediated drug-drug interactions in which the antidepressant is the target rather than the cause of the interaction.
- Some antidepressants (eg, nefazodone) are converted into metabolites with clinically important effects.[103,139]
- Difference in half-lives of the various antidepressants.[103,176] This issue is arguably the single most important pharmacokinetic difference among antidepressants beyond their effect on CYP enzymes.

TABLE 6.9 — EFFECT OF CYTOCHROME P450 ENZYMES ON SPECIFIC DRUGS (IE, METABOLISM)

CYP 1A2	
Antidepressants	Amitriptyline, clomipramine, imipramine
Antipsychotics	Clozapine,* olanzapine,* thioridazine*
β-Blockers	Propanolol
Opiates	Methadone*
Miscellaneous	Caffeine,* paracetamol, tacrine,* theophylline,* R-warfarin*
CYP 2C9/10	Phenytoin,* S-warfarin,* tolbutamide*
CYP 2C19	
Antidepressants	Citalopram,* clomipramine, imipramine
Barbiturates	Hexobarbital, mephobarbital, S-mephenytoin*
β-Blockers	Propranolol
Benzodiazepines	Diazepam

CYP 2D6	
Antiarrhythmics	Encainide,* flecainide,* mexiletine, propafenone
Antipsychotics	Haloperidol (minor), molindone, perphenazine,* risperidone,* thioridazine (minor)
β-Blockers	Alprenolol, bufuralol, metoprolol,* propranolol, timolol
Miscellaneous	Debrisoquine,* 4-hydroxyamphetamine, perhexiline,* phenformin, sparteine*
Opiates	Codeine,* dextromethorphan,* ethylmorphine
SSRIs	Fluoxetine, N-desmethylcitalopram, paroxetine*
TCAs	Amitriptyline,* clomipramine,* desipramine,* imipramine,* N-desmethylclomipramine
Other antidepressants	Venlafaxine,* mCPP metabolite of nefazodone* and trazodone*
CYP 3A3/4	
Analgesics	Acetaminophen, alfentanil
Antiarrhythmics	Amiodarone, disopyramide, lidocaine, propafenone, quinidine
Anticonvulsants	Carbamazepine,* ethosuximide
Antidepressants	Amitriptyline, clomipramine, imipramine, nefazodone,* sertraline,* O-desmethylvenlafaxine*

30%

50%

6

Continued

CYP 3A3/4 (continued)	
Antiestrogens	Docetaxel, paclitaxel, tamoxifen*
Antihistamines	Astemizole,* loratadine,* terfenadine*
Antipsychotics	Quetiapine,* clozapine
Benzodiazepines	Alprazolam,* clonazepam, diazepam, midazolam,* triazolam*
Calcium channel blockers	Diltiazem,* felodipine,* minodipine, nicardipine, nifedipine,* niludipine, nisoldipine, nitrendipine, verapamil*
Immunosuppressants	Cyclosporine,* tacrolimus (FK506-macrolide)
Local anesthetics	Cocaine, lidocaine
Macrolide antibiotics	Clarithromycin, erythromycin, triacetyloleandomycin
Steroids	Androstenedione, cortisol,* dehydro-3-epiandrosterone, dexamethasone, estrogen,* testosterone,* estradiol,* ethinylestradiol, progesterone
Miscellaneous	Benzphetamine, cisapride,* dapsone,* lovastatin, omeprazole (sulfonation)

Abbreviations: CYP, cytochrome P450 enzyme; SSRI, selective serotonin reuptake inhibitor; TCA, tricyclic antidepressants; mCPP, meta-chlorophenylpiperazine.

* Principal CYP enzyme.

NOTE: Such lists are not comprehensive since the CYP enzyme(s) responsible for biotransformation is known for only approximately 20% of marketed drugs. The reason is that many drugs were developed before the necessary knowledge and technology existed. Some drugs are listed under more than one CYP enzyme. That does not necessarily mean that each of these enzymes contributes equally to the elimination of the drug. One enzyme may be principally responsible based on substrate affinity and capacity and abundance of the enzyme.

Adapted from: Preskorn SH. *Clinical Pharmacology of Selective Serotonin Reuptake Inhibitors.* Caddo, Okla: Professional Communications, Inc; 1996:158-159.

6

TABLE 6.10 — The Inhibitory Effect of Newer Antidepressants at Their Usually Effective Minimum Dose on Specific CYP Enzymes

	No or Minimal Effect (< 20%)*	Mild (20%-50%)*	Moderate (50%-150%)*	Substantial (> 150%)*
Citalopram	1A2, 2C9/10, 2C19, 3A3/4	2D6	—	—
Fluoxetine	1A2	3A3/4	2C19	2D6, 2C9/10
Fluvoxamine	2D6	—	3A3/4	1A2, 2C19
Nefazodone	1A2, 2C9/10, 2C19, 2D6	—	—	3A3/4
Paroxetine	1A2, 2C9/10, 2C19, 3A3/4	—	—	2D6
Sertraline	1A2, 2C9/10, 2C19, 3A3/4	2D6	—	—
Venlafaxine	1A2, 2C9/10, 2C19, 3A3/4	2D6	—	—

Mirtazapine based on *in vitro* modeling is unlikely to produce clinically detectable inhibition of these five cytochrome P450 (CYP) enzymes. However, no *in vivo* studies have been done to confirm that prediction.

* Percent increase in plasma levels of a coadministered drug dependent on this CYP enzyme for its clearance.

Adapted from: Harvey A, Preskorn SH. *J Clin Psychopharmacol.* 1996;16:273-285, 345-355; Preskorn S. *Clinical Pharmacology of Selective Serotonin Reuptake Inhibitors.* Caddo, Okla: Professional Communications, Inc; 1996:176; and Shad MU, Preskorn SH. In: Levy R, et al, eds. Philadelphia, Pa; Lippincott, Williams & Wilkins. In press.

The Clinical Importance of Half-Life

Half-life is the time needed to decrease plasma drug concentration by 50% after drug discontinuation. As a general rule, steady-state is achieved when the drug has been administered at a stable dose for a period equal to 5 times its half-life. The same is true for washout following drug discontinuation. Thus, half-life is an important determinant of how long it will take to achieve maximal drug effect once started, and how long the effect will persist once the drug is stopped.[175]

The optimal dosing schedule for antidepressants is virtually never established empirically. Instead, the half-life is almost always used to determine the dosage schedule for a drug in the clinical trials required for its registration. That is done to maximize the chance for showing acceptable efficacy and tolerability. Since the FDA requires that the dosing schedules in the package inserts be based on the schedules used in the clinical trials, that means the half-life of the drug determines the recommended dosing schedule contained in the package insert.

In general, the half-life of most antidepressants is approximately 24 hours. For this reason, most of these drugs were administered once a day during clinical trials.[103,176] For the same reason, steady-state and virtually complete washout are achieved within 5 days of starting or stopping most of the newer antidepressants.

A few antidepressants have half-lives shorter than 24 hours including:

- Bupropion (Wellbutrin)
- Fluvoxamine (Luvox)
- Nefazodone (Serzone)
- Venlafaxine.[103] (Effexor)   SNRI

TABLE 6.11 — SUMMARY OF FORMAL *IN VIVO* STUDIES OF THE EFFECTS OF DIFFERENT SSRIS ON CYP 2D6 MODEL SUBSTRATES

SSRI	Author	N	SSRI Treatment: Dose (mg/day) × Duration (days)	Substrate	Substrate Dosing	Results (AUC2 – AUC1) ÷ AUC1*	DM/DO*	EMs to PMs
Citalopram	Gram	8	40 × 10	DMI	Single dose	47%		
Fluoxetine	Lam	8	60 × 8†	DM	Single dose		3484%	62.5%
	Amchin	12	20 × 28†	DM	Single dose		1711%	
	Bergstrom	6	60 × 8†	DMI	Single dose	640%		
	Bergstrom	6	60 × 8†	IMI	Single dose	IMI 235% DMI 430%		
	Preskorn	9	20 × 21	DMI	21 days	380%		
	Otton	19	37 ± 17 × 21	DM	Single dose			95%
	Mace	11	20 × 28	mCPP	7 days	820% (270%)‡		
Fluvoxamine	Lam	6	100 × 8	DM	Single dose		> 6%	0%
	Spina	6	100 × 10	DMI	Single dose	14%		

Paroxetine	Alderman	17	20 × 9	DMI	9 days	421%		
	Brosen	9	20 × 8	DMI	Single dose	364%		78%
	Albert	10	30 × 4	IMI	Single dose	IMI 74% DMI 327%		
	Lam	8	20 × 8	DM	Single dose		3943%	50%
	Ozdemir	8	20 × 10	PRZ	Single dose	595%		
Sertraline	Alderman	17	50 × 9	DMI	8 days	37%		
	Jann	4	50 × 7	DMI	7 days	0%		
	Preskorn	9	50 × 21	DMI	21 days	23%		
	Solai	13	50 × > 5	NTP	Chronic dosing	14%		
	Ozdemir	19	94 ± 26 × 24 ± 17	DM	Single dose	0%		0%
	Sproule	6	108 ± 49 × 21	DM	Single dose	5%	22%	0%
	Lam	7	100 × 8	DM	Single dose		28%	0%
	Kurtz	6	150 × 8	IMI	Single dose	68%		
		6	150 × 8	DMI	Single dose	54%		
	Zussman	13	150 × 29	DMI	Single dose	70%		

Continued

6

Abbreviations: SSRI, serotonin selective reuptake inhibitor; CYP, cytochrome P450 enzyme; AUC2, area under the curve of the substrate with SSRI; AUC1, area under the curve of the substrate without SSRI; DM, dextromethorphan; DO, dextrorphan; EM, extensive metabolizer; PM, poor metabolizer; DMI, desipramine; IMI, imipramine; mCPP, meta-chlorophenylpiperazine (a metabolite of nefazodone and trazodone); PRZ, perphenazine; NTP, nortriptyline.

* Percent increase.

† 60 mg/day for 8 days is a loading-dose strategy used to approximate the plasma levels of fluoxetine and norfluoxetine achieved under steady-state conditions on a dose of 20 mg/day.

‡ 820% is based on all the data. If the two highest increases are excluded, the average was 270%.

Adapted from: Preskorn SH. *J Psychopharmacology.* 1998;12:S89-S97.

For this reason, these drugs were tested using either a twice-a-day or even a three-times-a-day schedule during registration trials.

Since frequent dosing schedules are perceived as a disadvantage, extended-release formulations of bupropion and venlafaxine have been developed. Although the half-life of the drug remains the same, the extended absorption of these formulations produce reasonably stable blood levels of the drug over a more prolonged dosing interval.

The only antidepressant with a half-life substantially in excess of 24 hours is fluoxetine. The parent drug has a half-life of 2 to 4 days and norfluoxetine, its active metabolite, has a half-life of 7 to 15 days.[170] This half-life is even longer at doses above 20 mg/day in physically healthy older patients.[197] These half-lives mean that fluoxetine is essentially an oral depot drug that requires more than a month to:

- Reach steady-state once started
- Clear once stopped.

The practitioner must realize that once fluoxetine has achieved steady state, its effects cannot rapidly be reversed and that there will be an appreciable interval after its discontinuation during which fluoxetine (or norfluoxetine) can affect the response of the patient to other drug treatment, either through blockade of the serotonin uptake pump or through the inhibition of specific CYP enzymes (Chapter 10).

Antidepressant Withdrawal Syndrome

A general rule in clinical psychopharmacology is that the brain adapts to the presence of drugs. For example, uptake inhibitors produce downregulation of the receptors for the specific neurotransmitter whose uptake pump has been inhibited (eg, some serotonin receptors in the case of serotonin uptake inhibitors and beta-adrenergic receptors in the case of norepinephrine uptake inhibitors).[17] In fact, such downregulation has been postulated to mediate the antidepressant efficacy of these drugs.

Such downregulation likely also mediates the withdrawal syndromes that can be seen when some of these antidepressants are abruptly stopped. Anticholinergic withdrawal syndrome can be seen when high-potency muscarinic cholinergic receptor blockers (ie, TATCAs) are abruptly stopped. The symptoms of anticholinergic withdrawal syndromes (sometimes called "cholinergic rebound") are listed in Table 6.12.

The SRI withdrawal syndrome can be seen when serotonin uptake inhibitors are stopped (Table 6.13).[26,38,53,78,125,126,128,133,198,209,210,219,229,272] The SRI with-

---

TABLE 6.12 — SYMPTOMS OF ANTICHOLINERGIC WITHDRAWAL SYNDROME

- Loose stools
- Urinary frequency
- Headache
- Hypersalivation

TABLE 6.13 — SYMPTOMS OF SEROTONIN REUPTAKE INHIBITOR WITHDRAWAL SYNDROME

Serotonin reuptake inhibitor withdrawal syndrome can be remembered by using the mnemonic FLUSH:

- **F**lu-like:
  - Fatigue
  - Myalgia
  - Loose stools
  - Nausea
- **L**ightheadedness/dizziness
- **U**neasiness/restlessness
- **S**leep and sensory disturbances
- **H**eadache

drawal syndrome is more clinically important than is the anticholinergic withdrawal syndrome because it is more common, more severe, and more easily misdiagnosed. It can mimic worsening of the underlying depression or even as the emergence of mania. Such misdiagnosis can lead to inappropriate treatment.[38,125,126,128,209,210] The diagnosis is confirmed when the symptoms remit (typically within 12 to 24 hours) after restarting the SRI. After that, a more gradual taper can be done to wean the patient off the drug.

Risk factors for antidepressant withdrawal syndromes are:

- Time on drug
- Potency of drug
- Half-life of drug.[53,198,209]

As mentioned above, the shorter the half-life, the more likely the drug will wash out before the brain has had an opportunity to re-equilibrate (eg, upregulation of receptors) and, hence, the more likely that withdrawal symptoms will occur after drug discontinuation. Thus, the order of likelihood of the SRI withdrawal syndrome following abrupt discontinuation of an SRI is:

fluvoxamine, paroxetine, and venlafaxine > citalopram and sertraline, > fluoxetine.[53,198,209,219] The SRI withdrawal syndrome rarely occurs after nefazodone discontinuation.

Paroxetine and nefazodone deserve additional comment since the risk of an SRI withdrawal syndrome does not appear to correlate with their half-lives. In the case of paroxetine, the incidence of the SRI withdrawal syndrome is higher than might be expected for a drug with a half-life of 24 hours. However, the half-life of paroxetine is a function of its plasma levels. At low levels, the half-life of paroxetine is only 10 hours (ie, shortest of all the SRIs) due to the fact that it is preferentially metabolized by CYP 2D6 at low levels.[93,94,170] CYP 2D6 is a high-affinity, but low-capacity, enzyme for the metabolism of paroxetine and is inhibited by paroxetine. For this reason, this CYP enzyme becomes saturated at therapeutic levels of paroxetine (ie, autoinhibition), and CYP 3A3/4 becomes the primary mechanism for its elimination. CYP 3A3/4 is a low-affinity, but high-capacity, enzyme and hence produces a paroxetine half-life of 24 hours. When paroxetine is discontinued, its clearance accelerates as its level falls, and that likely accounts for the increased likelihood of an SRI withdrawal syndrome following its discontinuation.

In the case of nefazodone, the incidence of an SRI withdrawal syndrome is less than might be expected given its short half-life of 4 hours. There are several possible explanations that are not mutually exclusive:

- Nefazodone has several active metabolites which may cushion the withdrawal state, particularly the triazoledione metabolite, which has a considerably longer half-life than the parent drug, nefazodone.[103]
- Nefazodone is relatively weak as an SRI. Its most potent action is 5-HT2A blockade, which does not appear to cause a withdrawal liabil-

ity. In fact, pharmacologically relevant serotonin uptake inhibition requires a daily dose of nefazodone of at least 500 mg/day and possibly more.[150]

Either of these reasons may account for why patients treated with nefazodone at doses below 500 mg/day have a minimal risk of experiencing the SRI withdrawal syndrome following its discontinuation.

7

Considerations When
Selecting an Antidepressant

As a basis for conceptualizing the pharmacology of the 22 different antidepressant options available in the United States, Chapter 6 presented a classification system which grouped all available antidepressants into eight mechanistically defined classes. This chapter will translate that basic pharmacology into five clinically relevant factors to be considered when selecting any drug for any patient:

- **S**afety
- **T**olerability
- **E**fficacy
- **P**ayment
- **S**implicity.

These five factors are summarized by the mnemonic, **STEPS**. Each factor can be further subdivided as shown in Table 7.1. The discussion in this chapter will focus on each factor and present a summary of how each antidepressant group relates to that factor. A summary of the clinical pharmacology of each class of antidepressants as they relate to these five factors will be discussed in Chapter 8. A summary of how the various classes (and individual members within these classes) compare on these five factors is provided in Tables 7.2 through 7.9.

Safety

■ Acute Therapeutic Index

Tertiary amine tricyclic antidepressants (TATCAs) have a narrow acute therapeutic index due to their in-

TABLE 7.1 — STEPS CRITERIA FOR SELECTING AN ANTIDEPRESSANT

Safety
- Therapeutic index
- Drug-drug interactions:
  - Pharmacodynamics
  - Pharmacokinetics

Tolerability

Efficacy
- Overall
- Unique spectrum of activity
- Rate of response
- Maintenance and prophylaxis

Payment

Simplicity
- Ease of administration

Adapted from: Preskorn SH. *J Clin Psychiatry*. 1994;55(suppl A):6-22, 23-24, 98-100.

hibition of sodium (Na⁺) fast channels at concentrations only 10 times higher than those needed to treat major depression.[194] For this reason, an overdose of these drugs carries a serious risk of slowing intracardiac conduction to the point of inducing a fatal ventricular arrhythmia. This effect also occurs with secondary amine TCAs (eg, desipramine) even though these antidepressants are norepinephrine selective reuptake inhibitors (NSRIs) at usual therapeutic concentrations (Table 6.2). Other than TCAs, fatal overdose is not an issue with any other antidepressant when taken alone since they do not affect intracardiac conduction.

Some clinicians mistakenly believe that the arrhythmia caused by antidepressants such as desipramine is due to their ability to inhibit the neuronal uptake pump for norepinephrine. However, reboxetine (an investigational non-TCA NSRI) and venlafaxine (a serotonin and norepinephrine reuptake

106

TABLE 7.2 — STEPS CRITERIA FOR MIXED REUPTAKE AND NEURORECEPTOR ANTAGONISTS (EG, AMITRIPTYLINE) (Elavil)

Safety
- Therapeutic index: NARROW. Serious toxicity can result from overdose, either acute ingestion or from gradual accumulation due to slow clearance
- Drug-drug interactions:
  - Pharmacodynamic: prone to cause multiple types of such interactions due to their multiple mechanisms of action (Table 6.3)
  - Pharmacokinetic: can be the target of such interactions but are not prone to cause them. Due to narrow therapeutic index, care should be taken when prescribing TCAs to patients on drugs known to inhibit CYP enzymes (Table 6.10)

Tolerability
- Poor due to numerous types of adverse effects mediated by the blockade of histamine receptors (eg, sedation), muscarinic acetylcholine receptors (eg, constipation), and alpha-1–adrenergic receptors (eg, orthostatic hypotension) (Tables 6.2, 6.3, and 6.7)

Efficacy
- Overall: highest response rates of any antidepressants. Clomipramine in particular has been found to be superior to two SSRIs, citalopram and paroxetine, in hospitalized patients with clinical depression
- Unique spectrum of activity: imipramine has been found effective in patients who have not benefited from treatment with the SSRI, sertraline
- Rate of response: 2 to 4 weeks
- Maintenance of response: established by controlled studies

Payment
- Generic versions are available making these antidepressants the least expensive in terms of acquisition costs. These savings are likely offset by expenses arising from problems with their safety and tolerability (Table 7.10)

Simplicity
- Must titrate dose due to tolerability problems. Therapeutic drug monitoring should be done once early in treatment to guide dose adjustment. Therapeutic ranges have been established for most of these TCAs. Can be given once a day

Abbreviations: TCA, tricyclic antidepressant; CYP, cytochrome P450 enzyme; SSRI, serotonin selective reuptake inhibitor.

TABLE 7.3 — STEPS CRITERIA FOR NOREPINEPHRINE SELECTIVE REUPTAKE INHIBITORS (EG, DESIPRAMINE)*Norpramine*

Safety
- Therapeutic index: NARROW. The only NSRIs available at present in the United States are secondary amine TCAs which have the same toxicity problems as tertiary amine TCAs (eg, amitriptyline). However, this safety problem is due to inhibition of fast sodium channels as opposed to norepinephrine reuptake inhibition. In fact, there are investigational, nontricyclic NSRIs (eg, reboxetine) which do not have a narrow therapeutic index in terms of cardiotoxicity
- Drug-drug interactions:
  - Pharmacodynamic: limited at therapeutic concentrations to those produced by norepinephrine potentiation
  - Pharmacokinetic: can be target of such interactions but not prone to cause them. Due to narrow therapeutic index, care should be taken when prescribing with drugs known to inhibit CYP enzymes (Table 6.10)

Tolerability
- Generally good. Adverse effects mediated by norepinephrine potentiation (Tables 6.2, 6.3, and 6.6)

Efficacy
- Overall: comparable to tertiary amine TCAs
- Unique spectrum of activity: have been found in several studies to be effective in approximately 50% of patients who have not benefited from treatment with a variety of SSRIs
- Rate of response: 2 to 4 weeks
- Maintenance of response: established by controlled studies

Payment
- Generic versions are available but cost almost as much as newer antidepressants (Table 7.10)

Simplicity
- Can start on an effective dose immediately. Therapeutic drug monitoring should be done once early in treatment to guide dose adjustment. Therapeutic ranges have been established for most of these TCAs. Can be given once a day

Abbreviations: NSRI, norepinephrine selective reuptake inhibitor; TCA, tricyclic antidepressant; CYP, cytochrome P450 enzyme; SSRI, serotonin selective reuptake inhibitor.

TABLE 7.4 — STEPS CRITERIA FOR SEROTONIN SELECTIVE REUPTAKE INHIBITORS (EG, SERTRALINE)

Safety
- Therapeutic index: WIDE. No serious systemic toxicity demonstrated, even after substantial overdose
- Drug-drug interactions:
  - Pharmacodynamic: serotonin syndrome may occur when used with other serotonin agonists. Can potentiate dopamine antagonists in terms of extrapyramidal effects (eg, motor restlessness)
  - Pharmacokinetic: considerable differences exist among SSRIs in terms of their potential for decreasing the rate of oxidative metabolism of a variety of drugs by inhibiting CYP enzymes: fluoxetine, fluvoxamine > paroxetine > citalopram, sertraline (Table 6.10). No known clinically significant effect of other drugs on the clearance of SSRIs

Tolerability
- Good. Nausea and loose stools can occur early and are dose dependent but tolerance typically develops. Sexual dysfunction (eg, anorgasmia) can occur in approximately 30% of patients (Tables 6.2, 6.3, and 6.6)

Efficacy
- Overall: equivalent to TCAs in outpatients
- Unique spectrum of activity: can work in TCAs nonresponders
- Rate of response: 2 to 4 weeks
- Maintenance of response: evidence from controlled studies

Payment
- Brand name only available; see discussion (Table 7.10)

Simplicity
- Ease of administration: fluoxetine, paroxetine, and sertraline can be started at an effective dose immediately. Nonlinear pharmacokinetics of paroxetine likely contribute to an increased risk of experiencing an SRI discontinuation syndrome after abrupt cessation. The long half-life of fluoxetine and active metabolite, norfluoxetine, means time to maximum effect and time to washout can take up to 2 months

Abbreviations: SSRI, serotonin selective reuptake inhibitor; CYP, cytochrome P450 enzyme; TCA, tricyclic antidepressant; SRI, serotonin reuptake inhibitor.

TABLE 7.5 — STEPS CRITERIA FOR SEROTONIN AND NOREPINEPHRINE REUPTAKE INHIBITORS (EG, VENLAFAXINE)

Safety
- Therapeutic index: WIDE. No serious systemic toxicity demonstrated. Dose-dependent hypertension going from 1% above placebo at doses $\leq$ 100 mg/day to 11% above placebo at doses $\geq$ 300 mg/day. That fact is consistent with NE uptake inhibition occurring at higher doses
- Drug-drug interaction:
  – Pharmacodynamic: same as SSRIs at low doses. NE-mediated interactions possible at higher doses
  – Pharmacokinetic: has profile comparable to citalopram and sertraline in terms of no to minimal effects on most CYP enzymes (Table 6.10)

Tolerability
- Comparable to SSRIs at low dose; NE-mediated adverse effects at higher doses (Tables 6.2, 6.3, and 6.7)

Efficacy
- Overall: equivalent to TCAs. High-dose venlafaxine was superior to fluoxetine in double-blind study
- Unique spectrum of activity: possible efficacy in cases not responsive to TCAs or SSRIs
- Rate of response is a function of dose: 2 to 4 weeks at doses $\leq$ 150 mg/day and 4 to 7 days at doses of $\geq$ 300 mg/day
- Maintenance of response: evidence from controlled studies

Payment
- Brand name only available; see discussion (Table 7.10)

Simplicity
- Ease of administration: can be started at an effective dosage (75 mg/day); once daily dosing with sustained-release formulation. Dose titration is not necessary for many patients but increasing the dose is a reasonable strategy if starting dose is ineffective

Abbreviations: NE, norepinephrine; SSRI, serotonin selective reuptake inhibitor; CYP, cytochrome P450 enzyme; TCA, tricyclic antidepressant.

TABLE 7.6 — STEPS CRITERIA FOR SEROTONIN-2A RECEPTOR ANTAGONIST AND WEAK SEROTONIN REUPTAKE INHIBITORS (EG, NEFAZODONE)

Safety
- Therapeutic index: WIDE. No serious systemic toxicity due to acute overdose
- Drug-drug interactions:
  - Pharmacodynamic: can interact with other agents that decrease arousal or impair cognitive performance. Can interact with adrenergic agents affecting blood pressure regulation. Complex interactions with other serotonin-active agents
  - Pharmacokinetic: substantially inhibits CYP 3A which is responsible for 50% of known oxidative drug metabolism, including its own metabolism (ie, nonlinear pharmacokinetics or autoinhibition)

Tolerability
- Dizziness, drowsiness, and confusion are dose-dependent adverse effects; hence the need for dose titration (Tables 6.2, 6.3, and 6.7)

Efficacy
- Overall: equivalent to TCAs in outpatients
- Unique spectrum of activity: none demonstrated
- Rate of response: 2 to 4 weeks
- Maintenance of response: evidence from controlled studies

Payment
- Generic version of trazodone available. Brand name only for nefazodone. The latter has clinically important pharmacologic advantages over the former (Table 7.10)

Simplicity
- Ease of administration: requires dose titration and divided daily dosing for optimal antidepressant effect

Abbreviations: CYP, cytochrome P450 enzyme; TCA, tricyclic antidepressant.

TABLE 7.7 — STEPS CRITERIA FOR SEROTONIN (5-HT2A AND 5-HT2C) AND NOREPINEPHRINE (α-$_2$) RECEPTOR ANTAGONISTS (EG, MIRTAZAPINE) *Remeron*

Safety
- Therapeutic index: WIDE in terms of acute drug over-dose. There were three cases of agranulocytosis out of approximately 3000 patients in clinical trial program. That number was too small to establish with confidence the actual incidence or even whether there was a causal relation. Postmarketing experience has not indicated that toxicity is a major concern. Nevertheless, a white count should be obtained if a patient presents with signs of fever or infection
- Drug-drug interaction:
  – Pharmacodynamic: can cause multiple types of such interactions due to multiple mechanisms of action (Table 6.3)
  – Pharmacokinetic: unlikely to either be a victim or a cause of such interactions based on *in vitro* studies, but that should be confirmed by *in vivo* studies

Tolerability
- Primary problems are sedation due to histamine receptor blockade and weight gain due to 5-HT2C receptor blockade. These can be treatment limiting (Tables 6.2, 6.3, and 6.7). Dose titration may not help

Efficacy
- Overall: good; was superior to fluoxetine in double-blind study of hospitalized patients
- Unique spectrum of activity: worked in 54% of patients who had not benefited from treatment with amitriptyline. Open label studies have reported effectiveness in patients who had not benefited from SSRIs
- Rate of response: 2 to 4 weeks
- Maintenance of response: data limited to noncontrolled open label extension studies

Payment
- Brand name only available; see discussion (Table 7.10)

Simplicity
- Can start on an effective dose immediately. Sedation can be a problem, but starting with a lower dose may only decrease efficacy without improving tolerability, because mirtazapine is a more potent histamine receptor blocker than it is a serotonin and adrenergic receptor blocker. No rigorous data on whether higher doses increase either efficacy or tolerability

TABLE 7.8 — STEPS CRITERIA FOR DOPAMINE AND NOREPINEPHRINE REUPTAKE INHIBITORS (EG, BUPROPION) *Wellbutrin*

Safety
- Therapeutic index: NARROW. The dose needed for efficacy (300-450 mg/day) is only 2 to 3 times less than the dose that causes seizures in 2% of patients. That is the reason the maximum recommended daily dose is 450 mg/day. Seizures can also occur following an acute overdose but are generally managed easily in a medical setting
- Drug-drug interaction:
  - Pharmacodynamic: should potentiate and reduce the effects of other dopamine and norepinephrine agonists and antagonists, respectively
  - Pharmacokinetic: can be affected by fluoxetine and probably others in a clinically significant way. Due to its narrow therapeutic index, care should be taken when prescribing bupropion to patients on drugs known to inhibit CYP enzymes. Case report data suggest that it can substantially inhibit CYP 2D6

Tolerability
- Good. Does not cause sexual dysfunction seen with antidepressants which are serotonin reuptake inhibitors (Tables 6.2, 6.3, and 6.7)

Efficacy
- Overall: probably less than TCAs
- Unique spectrum of activity: can work in TCA nonresponders
- Rate of response: 2 to 4 weeks
- Maintenance of response: not demonstrated in formal studies

Payment
- Brand name only available; see discussion (Table 7.10)

Simplicity
- Ease of administration: requires divided daily dosing for antidepressant effect and dose titration to achieve efficacy and minimize seizure risk

Abbreviations: CYP, cytochrome P450 enzyme; TCA, tricyclic antidepressant.

TABLE 7.9 — STEPS CRITERIA FOR MONOAMINE OXIDASE INHIBITORS (EG, TRANYLCYPROMINE)

Safety
- Therapeutic index: NARROW. Serious toxicity can result from acute overdose
- Drug-drug interaction:
  - Pharmacodynamic: hypertensive crisis can result from coadministration with tyramine and sympathomimetic agents. Serotonin syndrome can result from coadministration with serotonin agonists (eg, serotonin uptake inhibitors) (Table 6.2)
  - Pharmacokinetic: inhibits the oxidative enzyme, MAOI, but effects on CYP enzymes have not been studied. Not known to be affected by other drugs in a clinically significant way

Tolerability
- Generally good, especially if kept to effective minimum dose. Ironically, main tolerability problem is hypotension (Table 6.3)

Efficacy
- Overall: Probably less than TCAs
- Unique spectrum of activity: can work in TCA nonresponders
- Rate of response: 2 to 4 weeks
- Maintenance of response: not adequately tested

Payment
- Generic versions are available making these antidepressants the least expensive in terms of acquisition costs (Table 7.10). These savings are likely offset by expenses arising from problems with their safety and tolerability

Simplicity
- Ease of administration: typically administered in divided daily doses. Dose titration recommended to optimize efficacy and minimize hypotension

Abbreviations: MAOI, monoamine oxidase inhibitor; CYP, cytochrome P450 enzyme; TCA, tricyclic antidepressant.

inhibitor [SNRI]) block norepinephrine uptake, but do not inhibit Na$^+$ fast channels even at concentrations achieved following a moderate overdose. Arrhythmias generally do not occur following overdose of these norepinephrine-active antidepressants.[41,73]

Although not as serious as the cardiotoxicity of TCAs, there are some safety concerns with some newer antidepressants. For example, bupropion has a dose-dependent risk of seizures.[57] At dosages of 450 mg/day, the seizure risk is 0.4%; that risk may be lower with the sustained-release formulations because of the blunting of peak levels. The risk of seizures due to bupropion increases substantially when its dosage exceeds 450 mg/day (the maximum recommended daily dosage).

Consistent with their pharmacology as indirect sympathomimetic agonists, NSRIs (eg, desipramine) and high-dosages of the SNRI venlafaxine (ie, > 225 mg/day) can cause dose-dependent increases in blood pressure.[73,169,240] The magnitude of the increases in blood pressure produced by these drugs is generally modest, but in some cases, can be sufficient to warrant either discontinuation or the addition of an antihypertensive medication.

Finally, some newer antidepressants (eg, fluoxetine) at their usually effective antidepressant dose produce substantial inhibition of one or more drug metabolizing cytochrome P450 (CYP) enzymes (Table 6.10 and Figure 6.2). That action carries with it the liability for causing clinically significant and even fatal pharmacokinetically mediated drug-drug interactions (Chapter 10).

■ Long-Term Safety
Antidepressants are among the most widely prescribed medications and are often taken on a long-term basis to prevent the recurrence of major depressive

episodes. There is no evidence of serious long-term safety problems with any antidepressant, based on spontaneous reports to the Food and Drug Administration (FDA). The long-term safety of antidepressants has also been systemically evaluated during clinical trial development programs.[103,169,178] The most rigorous data in this regard come from year-long, placebo-controlled relapse prevention studies.[62,67,112,148]

Other data come from open-label extension studies. In these studies, patients who have completed double-blind acute treatment studies can elect to continue on the medication until it is approved by the FDA. Given these two types of approaches, the safety of the drug will have typically been assessed in several hundred patients for up to 1 year by the time it is available in the United States.

■ Pharmacodynamic Interactions

The more sites of action affected by a drug, the more potential there is for pharmacodynamic interaction with other coprescribed drugs.[192] In fact, the sites of action affected by a drug determine the specific type of pharmacodynamic drug-drug interaction(s) it can cause.

Tertiary amine TCAs, due to their multiple effects on different neural targets (Table 6.2), will cause the most types of pharmacodynamic drug-drug interactions.[192] Specifically, these antidepressants can:

- Potentiate the sedative effects of alcohol and other sedative hypnotics via their blockade of the histamine-1 receptor
- Enhance the antiperistaltic effects of other drugs via their blockade of the muscarinic cholinergic receptor
- Increase the blood pressure-lowering effects of a variety of antihypertensives via their blockade of the alpha-1–adrenergic receptor

- Potentiate the slowing of intracardiac conduction produced by various antiarrhythmic agents via their inhibition of Na+ fast channels.
- Cause a hypertensive crisis when used with other norepinephrine agonists like monoamine oxidase inhibitors (MAOIs) due to their ability to inhibit the norepinephrine uptake pump
- Cause a serotonin syndrome when used with other serotonin agonists like MAOIs due to their ability to inhibit the serotonin uptake pump.

Using Tables 6.2 and 6.3, the clinician can determine which other antidepressants share the same potential to cause specific types of pharmacodynamic drug interactions as do the TATCAs.

■ Pharmacokinetic Interactions

The CYP enzyme-mediated drug-drug interactions are the most common type of pharmacokinetic drug-drug interaction.[93,94] The clinician can use Table 6.10 to determine which antidepressants are most likely to cause such interactions (ie, be the perpetrator). Table 6.9 can be used to determine which drugs will be affected (ie, be the victim) by an alteration (ie, induction or inhibition) in the metabolic capacity of a specific CYP enzyme. Fluoxetine and fluvoxamine will cause the most types of CYP enzyme-mediated drug interactions because they inhibit more than one CYP enzyme to a substantial degree at their usually effective antidepressant dose (Table 6.10 and Figure 6.2).

Pharmacokinetic drug interactions can present in many different ways (ie, decreased tolerability, decreased efficacy, withdrawal syndromes, or increased toxicity) because they typically produce an effect comparable to a change in the dose of the affected drug (Chapter 10). The clinician may not realize that starting or stopping the inhibitor has effectively changed the functional dose of the affected or victim drug by changing its clearance. Hence, the change in efficacy or tolerability may incorrectly be attributed to a patient sensitivity problem or to an underlying medical problem. Such misdiagnosis can:

- Prolong the patient's suffering
- Increase the cost of health care
- Complicate prescriber's management of patient.

Tolerability

■ Acute Tolerability Problems

As with drug-drug interactions, the more sites of action that a drug affects, the more types of adverse effects it can produce. The clinician can use Tables 6.2 and 6.3 to predict the types of adverse effects of each class of antidepressant. Tables 6.4 through 6.7 contain frequency of specific adverse effects for various antidepressants based on double-blind, placebo-controlled studies. Chapter 11 discusses the possible management approaches to the most common nuisance adverse effects of specific antidepressants.

■ Long-Term Tolerability Problems

Although most of the adverse effects caused by antidepressants occur after the first dose, or at least within the first week of treatment, sexual dysfunction is an exception.[145,147] This effect frequently does not come to clinical attention until several weeks or months into treatment. All antidepressants that produce substantial serotonin uptake inhibition can cause:

- Anorgasmia
- Decreased libido
- Delayed ejaculation.[145,147]

There is no universally effective treatment for the sexual dysfunction caused by serotonin uptake inhibitors, but potential useful "antidotes" are discussed in Chapter 11.

Other types of sexual dysfunction caused by antidepressants include:

- Tertiary amine TCAs can cause impotence via their alpha-1–adrenergic blockade.[103]
- Trazodone can cause priapism in approximately 1 in 8000 males.[103]

Norepinephrine uptake inhibitors (eg, *(Norpramine)* desipramine), *(Wellbutrin)* bupropion, *(Remeron)* mirtazapine and *(Serzone)* nefazodone at dosages below 500 mg/day appear to have minimal risk of causing sexual adverse effects.[103,151,171,213]

Efficacy

As with many other illnesses, the treatment of clinical depression can be divided into several clinically important and distinct phases as follows:

- Acute induction of remission
- Maintenance of remission during the vulnerable period of time for a relapse
- Prophylactic treatment to protect against future depressive episodes.[4,61,98]

There are several factors that need to be weighed when considering the induction of an acute remission as follows:

- Overall efficacy
- Unique spectrum of efficacy
- Rate of response.[169]

Clinical depression is a syndrome that will likely prove to be more than one illness when understood from the perspective of pathophysiology and/or etiology. The results of genetic and familial studies, biological marker studies, psychosocial studies and antidepressant clinical trials are all consistent with the conclusion that clinical depression is a heterogeneous group of disorders. That means that antidepressants with different mechanisms of action may treat different types of clinical depression (ie, have different overall acute efficacy and different spectra of efficacy).

Overall acute efficacy refers to how many patients with clinical depression will respond to a trial of a particular antidepressant. Assuming all other factors are equal (ie, safety, tolerability, cost and simplicity), the antidepressant of first choice would be the one that will produce a clinically meaningful, acute response in the largest number of patients.

Unique spectrum of efficacy refers to whether an antidepressant will work in a patient who has not benefited from a previous trial of another antidepressant. This issue is clinically important because virtually any antidepressant fails to produce an adequate response in one third to one half of patients suffering from clinical depression.

Rate of response is self-explanatory. This issue is more of interest to psychiatrists than to the primary-care practitioner, since the usual time course for response to an antidepressant (ie, approximately 2 weeks) does not typically pose a significant problem for outpatients with mild-to-moderate clinical depression.

Maintenance efficacy refers to whether there is evidence that continued treatment with the antidepressant is an effective strategy to prevent a relapse of the current episode. Since clinical depression is a recurrent condition in 50% or more of cases, *prophylactic efficacy* refers to whether there is evidence that indefinite treatment with an antidepressant in high-risk patients can prevent future episodes.

■ Overall Acute Efficacy

There is some evidence that drugs having more than one mechanism of antidepressant action may produce a higher percentage of response than do antidepressants with a single mechanism of action. Specifically, there are double-blind studies in which clomipramine (a TATCA), mirtazapine and venlafaxine produced a statistically significant better response rate than did an active control with a single mechanism of action (eg, serotonin uptake inhibition) in hospitalized patients with severe clinical depression.[48,55,56,267] On the other hand, antidepressants with multiple mechanisms of action often cause a higher dropout rate due to an increased incidence of adverse effects. Thus, their increased efficacy can be offset by the increased dropout rate such that the net outcome is a "wash."

■ Speed of Response

Most antidepressants take at least 2 weeks to demonstrate a higher response rate than the parallel placebo-controlled condition.[103] In fact, it is advisable to not give up on an antidepressant or even to increase the dose of the single-mechanism-of-action antidepressant until a trial of at least 4 weeks on a stable dose has been given. In contrast, there is one study indicating that high-dosage venlafaxine (ie, > 300 mg/day) can produce a response in 20% of patients within 1 week and can statistically separate from placebo as soon as 4 days.[169] These findings are consistent with combined inhibition of both serotonin and norepinephrine uptake pumps at such doses of venlafaxine (Figure 6.4).[103] A similar rapid onset of antidepressant action has also been produced by using a combination of an NSRI (eg, desipramine) and a serotonin selection reuptake inhibitor (SSRI) (eg, sertraline).[153,258]

Of course, either of these approaches (ie, high dose venlafaxine or combined use of an NSRI and an

121

SSRI) to increase efficacy by affecting these two mechanisms of action sets the stage for more types of adverse effects mediated by these two different mechanisms of action (Table 6.5). The increase in tolerability problems can more than offset the increase in efficacy, particularly in the primary-care setting where there is typically no need for a more rapid response than is achieved with conventional antidepressant treatment. Nevertheless, these strategies can be useful when dealing with a severely ill or hospitalized patient where time of response is a critical issue.

■ Unique Spectrum of Efficacy

One advantage of having eight mechanistically different classes of antidepressants is the possibility that patients who are intolerant of or do not respond to one type of antidepressant may benefit from treatment with a mechanistically different type of antidepressant. While this possibility is intuitively plausible, this subject has received scant systematic study (Chapter 11). Most studies that have tested this possibility have not been scientifically rigorous, but were instead open label and hence subject to potential biases.

The best data on this topic come from a series of double-blind, crossover studies with NSRIs and SSRIs.[245] Based on these studies, approximately 50% of patients who do not benefit from a trial of an SSRI will benefit when switched to an NSRI. The reverse is also true. This evidence is also fully consistent with the aforementioned data that combined treatment with an NSRI and an SSRI or with high-dose venlafaxine produces more responders than does treatment with either mechanism alone. While the available data are modest, there certainly is no evidence to suggest that a nonresponse to one type of antidepressant predicts nonresponse to a mechanistically different type of antidepressant.[61,245]

■ Maintenance and Prophylactic Efficacy

The FDA does not require proof of either maintenance or prophylactic efficacy to approve a drug as an antidepressant. Nevertheless, most approved newer antidepressants have been tested and shown to have sustained efficacy over the maintenance phase (ie, 6 months after the induction of an acute remission). The best studies involve open-label treatment for 2 to 3 months to induce an acute response and then double-blind, random assignment to either remain on the antidepressant or be switched to placebo.[62,67,148] Approximately one fourth to one third more patients on placebo will relapse back into their depressive episode over a 6-month interval in comparison to those maintained on the antidepressant. These data are sufficiently compelling so that continued treatment with an antidepressant for 6 months after an acute response is recommended for all first-episode patients.[4,61]

Less well studied is the issue of prophylactic efficacy. The single best study has been done with the TATCA, imipramine.[76] The follow-up treatment period for most patients in this study was 3 years, but some were followed for 5 years. The patients were selected for being at high risk for relapse. Participants were required to have had at least four episodes of depression (ie, the current one plus three prior episodes). The results provided compelling support for the benefit of prophylactic treatment with an antidepressant in such a high risk population—only 20% of the patients who remained on imipramine relapsed at the end of 3 years versus 95% of patients who were switched to placebo. A more recent 76-week, double-blind, randomized, parallel-group study demonstrated the superiority of sertraline over placebo in the maintenance treatment of patients with chronic major depression.[112]

Studies with other antidepressants have generally not lasted more than 1 year and have not been conducted in patients with such a high risk for recurrent episodes. Nevertheless, these studies have also demonstrated fewer recurrent episodes on drug versus a parallel, placebo-controlled condition.

Payment

This issue is complex, controversial, and not unique to antidepressants. Clinicians often find themselves between two competing forces:
- The pharmaceutical company, which develops a new medication
- The patient or their third-party insurer, who pays for the medication.

The latter is generally concerned with the acquisition cost (ie, how much does the prescription cost) (Table 7.10). The former points out that the increased acquisition cost of the new medication is more than offset by other "hidden" costs of the older and often generic drugs.

For example, the acquisition cost of a TATCA is considerably less than all of the newer antidepressants, but there are other associated costs that should be taken into account when doing a cost comparison.[40] These include but are not limited to:
- More physician visits
- Additional laboratory tests. For example, therapeutic drug monitoring should be done at least once when prescribing TCAs due to their narrow therapeutic index and high interindividual variability in clearance
- In the case of TCAs, there is also the cost of intensive care for the patient who takes an acute overdose
- Cost of treating adverse effects

• Tolerability problems may also have a hidden cost if the patient relapses because the medication was stopped too soon due to a persistent adverse effect.

Simplicity

An important issue when selecting an antidepressant is how easily can the clinician select an optimal dose for the patient; that is, determine the dose which has the greatest likelihood of producing a good antidepressant response and the least risk of causing either nuisance or serious adverse effects (Table 7.11).[169] This issue is particularly important for the primary-care practitioner given time constraints in daily practice.

A related issue is how easy is it for the patient to take the medication as prescribed. An ideal drug would be one that:

• Can be started at an effective dose (ie, no need for titration)
• Optimum dose easily determined
• Requires no special laboratory testing to guard against toxicity either before or during treatment
• Can be taken once daily.

■ Start At Effective Dose

Several of the antidepressants meet many of the requirements above. Most SSRIs (ie, fluoxetine, paroxetine, and sertraline, but not citalopram and fluvoxamine), mirtazapine, most NSRIs (eg, desipramine, nortriptyline), and venlafaxine can be started at an effective dose. A few additional comments are warranted with regard to mirtazapine. Sedation can be a problem in early treatment with mirtazapine.[178] For this reason, some clinicians may

125

TABLE 7.10 — AVERAGE WHOLESALE PRICE OF REPRESENTATIVE DOSES OF ANTIDEPRESSANTS*

Generic/Trade Drug Name	Strength (mg)	Price ($/100)	
		Generic	Trade
Tertiary Amine Tricyclic Antidepressants			
Amitriptyline/Elavil	25	10	40
	50	12	72
	100	18	125
Doxepin/Sinequan	25	14	47
	50	19	65
	100	40	119
Imipramine/Tofranil	25	6	47
	50	9	80
Selective Norepinephrine Reuptake Inhibitors			
Desipramine/Norpramin	25	25	65
	50	50	122
	100	100	204

Nortriptyline/Pamelor	25		80	100
	50		150	190
Serotonin Selective Reuptake Inhibitors				
Citalopram/Celexa	20		NA	193
	40		NA	202
Fluoxetine/Prozac	10		NA	230
	20		NA	240
Fluvoxamine/Luvox	50		NA	206
	100		NA	212
Paroxetine/Paxil	10		NA	190
	20		NA	200
	30		NA	210
	40		NA	222
Sertraline/Zoloft	50		NA	180
	100		NA	200

Continued

Generic/Trade Drug Name	Strength (mg)	Price ($/100)	
		Generic	Trade
Serotonin and Norepineprhine Reuptake Inhibitors			
Venlafaxine-IR/*Effexor IR*	37.5	NA	105[†]
	75	NA	115[†]
	100	NA	122[†]
Venlafaxine-XR/*Effexor XR*	37.5	NA	194
	75	NA	217
	150	NA	237
Serotonin 2A Antagonists			
Nefazodone/*Serzone*	100, 150, 200, 250	NA	93[†]
Trazodone/*Desyrel*	50	30	150
	100	40	250
	300	NA	390

Serotonin (5-HT2A and 2C) and Adrenergic (α-2) Antagonists			
Mirtazapine/Remeron	15	NA	195
	30	NA	202
Dopamine and Norepinephrine Reuptake Inhibitors			
Bupropion-IR/Wellbutrin IR	75	NA	60[†]
	100	NA	83[†]
Bupropion-SR/Wellbutrin SR	100	NA	115[†]
	150	NA	117[†]
Monoamine Oxidase Inhibitors			
Phenelzine/Nardil	15	NA	42
Tranylcypromine/Parnate	10	NA	50

Abbreviations: NA, none available; IR, immediate release; SR, sustained release; XR, extended release.

* Information taken from 1998 *Drug Topics Red Book* and rounded to the nearest dollar.

† Recommended dosing is twice or three times a day, whereas other drugs in this chart are given once a day. That difference will affect the daily cost of treatment (ie, how long 100 pills will last).

TABLE 7.11 — SUMMARY OF PACKAGE INSERT DOSING GUIDELINES

Generic/Trade Name	Recommended Dose Start/Max (mg/day)[a,b]	Dosage Guidelines for Specific Patients				
		Children	Adolescents	Elderly	Hepatic*	Renal*
Mixed Reuptake Inhibitors and Neuroreceptor Blockers[a,b]						
Amitriptyline/Elavil	75/300[c]	↓	NA		↓	↓
Amoxapine/Ascendin	100/600[c,d]	NR	NA	↓	↓	↓
Clomipramine/Anafranil[e]	25/250[c,f]	NA	NA	↓	↓	↓
Doxepin/Sinequan	75/300[c]	NA	NA	NA	↓	↓
Imipramine/Tofranil	75/300[c]	NA	↓	↓	↓	↓
Norepinephrine Selective Reuptake Inhibitors[a,b]						
Desipramine/Norpramin	100/300[c]	↓	NA	↓	↓	↓
Maprotiline/Ludiomil	75/225[c,f]	NA	NA	↓	↓	↓
Nortriptyline/Pamelor	50/150[c]	NA	NA	↓	↓	↓
Serotonin Selective Reuptake Inhibitors						
Citalopram/Celexa	20/60	NA	NA	↓	↓	↓
Fluoxetine/Prozac	20/80	NA	NA	↓	↓	↓

Fluvoxamine/Luvox[e]	50/300[g]	NR	NA	→	→	→
Paroxetine/Paxil	20/50	NA	NA	→	→	→
Sertraline/Zoloft	50/200	↓	Same	Same	→	→
Serotonin and Norepinephrine Reuptake Inhibitors						
Venlafaxine-IR/Effexor IR	75[g,h]/375[g]	NA	NA	NA	→	→
Venlafaxine-XR/Effexor XR	75[h]/375	NA	NA	NA	→	→
Serotonin (5-HT2A) Receptor Blockers and Weak Serotonin Uptake Inhibitors						
Nefazodone/Serzone	200[g]/600[g]	NA	NA	→	→	→
Trazodone/Dyserel	150[g]/600[g]	NA	NA	→	→	→
Serotonin (5-HT2A and 5-HT2C) and Norepinephrine Receptor Blockers						
Mirtazapine/Remeron	15/45	NA	NA	→	→	→
Dopamine and Norepinephrine Reuptake Inhibitors						
Bupropion-IR/Wellbutrin IR	200[g]/450[c,f,i]	NA	NA	→	→	→
Bupropion-SR/Wellbutrin SR	150/400[c,f,i]	NA	NA	→	→	→
Monoamine Oxidase Inhibitors						
Phenelzine/Nardil	45[g]/90[g]	NA	NA	→	→	→
Tranylcypromine/Parnate	30[g]/60[g]	NA	NA	→	→	→

7

Abbreviations: NA, not available; NR, not recommended; IR, immediate release; XR, extended release; SR, sustained release.

* Impairment.

a   Starting dose may be given either as a once-a-day dose or on a divided schedule. Once an effective and tolerated dose has been established, it may be given on a once-a-day basis, but a divided dose may still be more prudent with a higher total dose and in patients who are elderly or debilitated. The maximum once-a-day dose of doxepin is 150 mg.

b   Usual dose may be given either as a once-a-day dose or on a divided schedule.

c   Therapeutic drug monitoring has been either demonstrated to increase the safe and efficacious use of this drug or theoretically should; demonstrated for amitriptyline, clomipramine, desipramine, imipramine, and nortriptyline. Theoretical for the rest, but has not been adequately studied.

d   Doses should exceed 400 mg/day only in hospitalized patients who do not have a history of seizures and who have not benefited from an adequate trial of 400 mg/day.

e   Not formally labeled by the FDA for the treatment of clinical depression but rather for obsessive-compulsive disorder; labeled for use as an antidepressant in other countries.

f   Maximum daily dose should not be exceeded due to an increased risk of seizures.

g   Dose should be given on a divided schedule (bid or tid).

h   For some patients, it may be desirable to start at half the dose for 4 to 7 days to improve tolerance, particularly in terms of nausea.

i   It is particularly important to administer in a manner most likely to minimize the risk of seizures. Dose increases should not exceed 100 mg/day in a 3-day period. Cautious dose titration can also minimize agitation, motor restlessness, and insomnia. Time between doses should be at least 4 hours for 100 mg IR doses, 6 hours for 150 mg IR doses, and 8 hours for SR doses. Increases above 300 mg/day should only be done in patients with no clinical effects after several weeks of treatment at 300 mg/day. Bupropion should be discontinued in patients who do not experience an adequate response after an adequate period on maximum recommended daily dose. Dosing in the elderly, the debilitated, and patients with hepatic and/or renal impairment has not been adequately studied so increased caution may be prudent.

Additional comments on dose titration: The package inserts for the following drugs indicate that they can be started at a dose which is usually effective to treat clinical depression: fluoxetine, mirtazapine, paroxetine, tranylcypromine, sertraline, venlafaxine. The following comments apply about the use of higher doses with these antidepressants. *For fluoxetine, paroxetine, and sertraline:* although fixed-dose studies in patients with clinical depression found no advantage on average to higher doses, an increase may be considered after several weeks on the starting dose if no clinical improvement has been observed. *For mirtazapine,* dose escalation should not be made at intervals of less than 1 to 2 weeks to adequately evaluate therapeutic response to a given dose. *For tranylcypromine,* improvement can be seen between 48 hours and 2 weeks of starting therapy; if not, dose increases in 10 mg/day increments may be made at intervals of 1 to 3 weeks.

The package inserts for the following drugs recommend starting at a lower than usually effective dose and titrate up to a dose which is usually effective to treat clinical depression in order to minimize tolerability or safety problems: amitriptyline, amoxapine, bupropion, citalopram, clomipramine, fluvoxamine, doxepin, imipramine, nefazodone, phenelzine, trazodone, and trimipramine. The following are additional comments about dose titration with these antidepressants: *For the tricyclic antidepressants,* the dose should be gradually increased during the first 2 weeks based on therapeutic drug monitoring and clinical assessment of efficacy and tolerability. *For fluvoxamine,* a lower than usually effective starting dose is recommended to improve tolerability. The dose should be increased every 4 to 7 days as tolerated until maximum therapeutic benefit is achieved. *For citalopram,* the starting dose is 20 mg/day with the recommendation to generally increase to 40 mg/day. While doses above 40 mg/day are not ordinarily recommended, some patients may require a dose of 60 mg/day. *For nefazodone,* a lower than usually effective starting dose is recommended to improve tolerability. Dose titration should occur in increments of 100 to 200 mg/day as determined by tolerability and the need for further clinical improvement. These incremental advances should be done using divided doses and at intervals of at least 1 week. It may be advisable to titrate up more slowly in elderly and debilitated patients. *For phenelzine,* a lower than usually effective starting dose is recommended to improve tolerability. Its dose should be increased to at least 60 mg/day at a fairly rapid pace consistent with good tolerability. *For trazodone,* the same comments apply as for nefazodone when trazodone is used as an antidepressant; however, it is now mainly used as a nonhabit-forming sedative given as a single bedtime dose of 50 to 200 mg as needed for sleep.

7

133

consider starting with a lower dose (7.5 mg), but this strategy may not avoid sedation (the drug's most common effect [Table 6.7]) and may compromise efficacy.[151]

In contrast to the above antidepressants, bupropion, nefazodone, and TATCAs do require dose titration primarily to minimize adverse effects.[103] In the case of bupropion, the goal of titration is to find the lowest effective dose to minimize the risk of seizures.[57] In the case of nefazodone and TATCAs, the issue is minimizing nonserious but nevertheless nuisance and sometimes rate-limiting adverse effects.

■ Ease of Optimum Dosing

The next issue is how easily the optimal dose of the antidepressant can be determined. Therapeutic plasma level ranges have been established for most TCAs. Thus, the clinician can use therapeutic drug monitoring (TDM) to adjust the dosage to compensate for interindividual differences in clearance in order to optimize the likelihood of antidepressant efficacy while simultaneously avoiding toxicity.[191] While increasing efficacy is an advantage of TDM with TCAs, the principal and compelling reason to use TDM with TCAs is to avoid toxicity in slow metabolizers. This is not an issue with any other class of antidepressants with the possible exception of bupropion.[180]

In the case of the SSRI class, there is no advantage to using higher than the usually effective minimum dose.[170] This finding is based on the results of double-blind, fixed-dose studies which have found flat dose-response curves above the usually effective minimum dose for these antidepressants.[170] This finding does not preclude the possibility that some patients may benefit from a higher dose of an SSRI (Chapter 11). Although beyond the scope of this book, paroxetine is the only SSRI for which there is substantial evidence that higher doses are needed to treat patients with anxiety disorders versus patients with clinical depression. The reasons for this dosing difference are not clear.

In contrast to SSRIs, there is an ascending dose-antidepressant response curve with venlafaxine.[177] This antidepressant at its starting dosage of 75 mg/day produces approximately the same number of responders as do the SSRIs, but the percentage of responders increase with higher doses consistent with its apparent dual mechanism of antidepressant action (ie, serotonin and then norepinephrine uptake inhibition). Consistent with its pharmacology, higher doses of venlafaxine also cause a higher incidence of serotonin- and norepinephrine-mediated adverse effects, including the potential to increase blood pressure as previously discussed.

There are no published fixed-dose studies which empirically establish that doses of mirtazapine higher than 15 mg/day are more effective or better tolerated. There are anecdotal and theoretical reasons to suspect that higher doses will decrease the problem of sedation (ie, offsetting arousal effects as a result of alpha-2–adrenergic blockade at higher concentrations [Figure 6.4]). However, in the case of bupropion and nefazodone, the optimal dose in terms of efficacy and tolerability is quite variable and requires empiric dose titration.[103]

Most of the antidepressants can be given once a day. The exceptions are bupropion (including the sustained-release formulation) and nefazodone which require at least twice-a-day dosing (Table 7.11). While once-a-day dosing is desirable, the available literature suggests that problems with compliance do not become an issue until the required dosing frequency is 3 times a day or more.

8   Evaluating the Various Antidepressants

This chapter will review each of the eight mechanistically defined classes of antidepressants and summarize their safety, tolerability, efficacy, payment and simplicity (STEPS) characteristics specifying which are an advantage and disadvantages for that class. When there are clinically meaningful differences between members of a class, those differences will be highlighted. The goal is to present a synopsis of the clinically relevant pharmacology of these drugs to aid the practitioner in making the best choice for a specific clinically depressed patient, including the usual patient and also particular subtypes of patients.

This approach and information should aid the busy primary-care practitioner in medication selection, particularly considering only 7 minutes are often allocated for a patient visit. Current prescribing data indicates that the serotonin selective reuptake inhibitors (SSRIs) as a class are the antidepressants of first choice for most practitioners, with over 50% of all antidepressant prescriptions being for one of the five SSRIs (Table 8.1). While a review of STEPS is consistent with that general prescribing pattern, a review of the available data does not support the share of the market commanded by fluoxetine and paroxetine. Their numbers suggest that many prescribers do not understand the significant problems posed by the fact that these SSRIs are prone to cause clinically significant drug-drug interactions as a result of their inhibition of specific cytochrome P450 (CYP) enzymes and have no offsetting advantage when compared to SSRIs (ie, citalopram and sertraline) which do not have this

TABLE 8.1 — PERCENTAGE OF NEW PRESCRIPTIONS WRITTEN FOR SPECIFIC ANTIDEPRESSANTS DURING OCTOBER, 1998

Antidepressant	Prescription (%)
Mixed Uptake and Neuroreceptor Blockers (17.9)	
Amitriptyline	12.2
Doxepin	2.8
Imipramine	2.9
Norepinephrine Selective Reuptake Inhibitors (4.4)	
Desipramine	0.8
Nortriptyline	3.6
Serotonin Selective Reuptake Inhibitors (50.5)	
Citalopram	1.1
Fluoxetine	17.5
Fluvoxamine	1.2
Paroxetine	14.5
Sertraline	16.2
Serotonin and Norepinephrine Reuptake Inhibitors (5.0)	
Venlafaxine-XR	3.1
Venlafaxine-IR	1.9
Serotonin-2A Blockers* (12.0)	
Nefazodone	3.5
Trazodone	8.5
Specific Serotonin and Adrenergic Receptor Blocker† (1.9)	
Mirtazapine	1.9
Dopamine and Norepinephrine Reuptake Inhibitor (7.9)	
Bupropion-SR	6.3
Bupropion-IR	1.6
Monoamine Oxidase Inhibitors (< 0.1)	

Abbreviations: TCA, tricyclic antidepressant; XR, extended release; IR, immediate release; SR, sustained release.

* Also weakly inhibits the serotonin uptake pump.
† Most potent action is histamine receptor blockade.

disadvantage. Another interesting fact that emerges from the prescribing data is that tertiary amine tricyclic antidepressants (TATCAs) are the second most commonly prescribed class of antidepressants, representing 20% of antidepressant prescriptions. However, a number of the prescriptions for TATCAs may be for indications other than clinical depression (eg, chronic pain, migraine headache).

Nevertheless, the prescribing data indicates that SSRIs and TATCAs account for seven out of ten prescriptions for antidepressants in the United States. Thus, the other six classes account for only 30% of antidepressant prescriptions, suggesting that some clinicians may not be taking full advantage of all the antidepressant options available. The goal of this chapter is to summarize the clinically relevant pharmacology of each class (and individual members within each class as appropriate) to aid the busy practitioner in selecting the best option for a patient whether the patient:

- Has classic clinical depression or a special subtype of clinical depression (eg, atypical or bipolar depression)
- Is a first-time patient or whose depression has proven to be refractory to the first antidepressant selected
- Is medically healthy
- Is on multiple other medications due to intercurrent medical illness.

Mixed Reuptake Inhibitors and Neuroreceptor Blockers

■ Tertiary Amine Tricyclic Antidepressants

The chance discovery of the antidepressant properties of TATCAs and the monoamine oxidase inhibitors (MAOIs) began the modern era of antidepressant pharmacology almost 50 years ago.

Advantages

- Efficacy: No single class of antidepressants works in more patients than TATCAs.[103] Several studies have reported higher response rates in hospitalized, depressed patients treated with the TATCA clomipramine, than with the SSRIs, citalopram or paroxetine.[55,56] Clinical trials have also shown that TATCAs are effective in patients who have not benefited from a trial of an SSRI.[245]

- TATCAs are also useful in a variety of conditions other than clinical depression including:
  - Chronic pain
  - Migraine headaches
  - Insomnia.

  For these indications, practitioners often prescribe considerably lower doses which minimize both the adverse effects of these drugs and their overdose risk.

- Payment: Cost can be an advantage of these antidepressants when the choice is between being able to treat or not. That can occur when the patient's insurance does not cover the cost of medication and the patient has limited personal financial resources (Table 7.10).

- Simplicity of dosing: All of the TATCAs can be taken once a day.[103] Since therapeutic ranges have been established for these antidepressants, therapeutic drug monitoring (TDM) can be used to rationally guide dose adjustments to ensure the attainment of levels which produce the greatest likelihood of antidepressant response with minimal risk of adverse effect.[191]

Disadvantages

- Safety: TATCAs have a narrow therapeutic index. Even a moderate overdose (ie, taking a 1-to-2-week supply at once) can cause life-threatening cardiotoxicity.[194] This toxicity risk alone is sufficient reason to rule out members of this class as the preferred agent for most patients.

- The multiple actions of TATCAs also mean that these antidepressants can interact pharmacodynamically with a number of other types of drugs including:
  - Sedative hypnotics and alcohol
  - Antihypertensives
  - Antiarrhythmics
  - Anticholinergics.
- Tolerability: By virtue of their effects on various sites of action, these agents cause many different types of adverse effects. Also, the percentage of patients who report adverse effects on these antidepressants is considerably higher than on any other type of antidepressant (Table 6.7). Adverse effects can affect the patient's functioning at work and home. The sedation and orthostatic hypotension have been linked to the increased incidence of falls resulting in hip fractures and automobile accidents in patients taking TATCAs.[132,239] They can also cause or aggravate other medical conditions. For example, patients on chronic treatment with TATCAs also have an increased likelihood of developing periodontal disease as a result of the loss of the bacteriostatic effects of saliva.[4]
- Simplicity of dosing: Their multiple mechanisms of action also mean that most patients cannot be started on the usually effective antidepressant dose of these drugs. Instead, the dose must be gradually titrated up as the patient develops tolerance to the acute adverse effects of the TATCAs. This approach builds in a delay in terms of relief of the patient's depressive episode. Even with a gradual titration,

141

adverse effects generally persist to some degree and can include a trio of adverse effects including:

– Sedation due to histamine-1 blockade
– Dry mouth, constipation, urinary retention, and memory impairment due to cholinergic receptor blockade
– Orthostatic hypotension or dizziness due to alpha-1–adrenergic receptor blockade (Table 6.7).

Summary

Tertiary amine TCAs are not recommended as the antidepressant of first choice for the general patient. However, they can be quite helpful for specific patients but require careful dose adjustment. TDM is a standard of care issue when prescribing these antidepressants due to their narrow therapeutic index and the wide interindividual variability in patients' metabolism.[191] However, TDM generally is needed only once early in treatment to determine whether the patient is a usual, slow or rapid TCA metabolizer. The dose can then be adjusted to ensure the attainment of safe and effective drug concentrations. After that, TDM is only done for cause such as a significant change in the patient's health status, the addition or discontinuation of a drug (eg, fluoxetine) that could affect drug metabolism, or to confirm that the patient is being compliant with the prescription.

The principal reasons to use a TATCA are:

• Low acquisition cost (Table 7.10)
• Treatment refractory clinical depression
• Presence of a comorbid medical condition (eg, chronic pain) which is responsive to these medications.

Alyce.

In such instances, imipramine *Tofranil* is the generally preferred TATCA for several reasons. First, it is one of

142

the least expensive antidepressants in terms of acquisition cost (Table 7.10). Second, imipramine is converted in the body to the secondary amine TCA
(SATCA), desipramine.[188] In the usual patient on imipramine, 50% of the total circulating TCA level will
be desipramine. That percentage can be as high as
90% in rapid demethylators. This conversion is an
advantage because desipramine has the best tolerability profile of all of the SATCAs due to its selective
action on the norepinephrine uptake pump (Figure
6.1). The tolerability profile of desipramine is generally comparable to most newer antidepressants.

Nevertheless, 50% of patients will have over half
of their circulating TCA level be imipramine rather
than desipramine.[188] These patients will have the adverse effect profile associated with imipramine rather
than desipramine (Tables 6.5 and 6.7). The practitioner can use TDM to establish whether the patient
achieves predominantly high levels of desipramine or
imipramine. In the case of slow demethylators who
accumulate high levels of imipramine relative to desipramine, the clinician may decide to switch to desipramine if there are significant tolerability problems
with imipramine. Unfortunately, the cost of desipramine is not appreciably less than many of the
newer antidepressants (Table 7.10).

Norepinephrine Selective Reuptake Inhibitors

■ Secondary Amine Tricyclic Antidepressants

The SATCAs are structural analogues of the
TATCAs. While they were not rationally developed
in the same way as the SSRIs, they were developed
because they had less antihistaminergic and less anticholinergic effects in animal models than did their
TATCA forerunners (Figure 6.1). They also do not
potently block alpha-1–adrenergic receptors. At usual

therapeutic concentrations, these antidepressants only block the norepinephrine uptake pump which is the presumed mechanism mediating their antidepressant efficacy (Table 6.2). Their clinical advantages and disadvantages stem directly from their pharmacology.

Advantages

- Safety: In comparison to TATCAs, these antidepressants have less potential for causing pharmacodynamic drug-drug interactions being limited to those mediated by norepinephrine uptake inhibition (eg, hypertensive crisis when combined with other norepinephrine agonists, particularly MAOIs).
- Tolerability: The discontinuation rate because of adverse effects on SATCAs is comparable to that of newer antidepressants, including SSRIs. Given their different mechanism of action, the adverse effects produced by these antidepressants are different from SSRIs. For that reason, they are an option for the patient who does not tolerate the adverse effects produced by SSRIs (Tables 6.4 and 6.6). The most common adverse effects on SATCAs are those expected for drugs that are indirect noradrenergic agonists, including:
  - Mild increase in blood pressure
  - Increased diaphoresis
  - Tachycardia
  - Tremors
  - Anxiety.[88]
- Efficacy: They are as effective as any other class of antidepressants, and double-blind, crossover studies have shown them to be effective in 50% of patients who do not benefit from treatment with an SSRI.[245] They can also be added to SSRIs to augment partial response or to speed response when clinically necessary (ie,

hospitalized patient). This strategy produces dual serotonin and norepinephrine uptake inhibition as occurs with high-dose ven-lafaxine.[177] The difference is that the use of an SSRI and a norepinephrine selective reuptake inhibitor (NSRI) together allows the dose (and hence the degree of uptake inhibition) of either one to be adjusted independently of the other. In contrast, a dual reuptake inhibitor like venlafaxine is analogous to a fixed combination of an SSRI and an NSRI and, thus, the relative ratio of the uptake inhibition of serotonin and norepineprhine is also fixed.

- Simplicity of dosing: All of the SATCAs can be taken once a day. Since therapeutic ranges have been established for these antidepressants, TDM can be used to rationally guide dose adjustment to ensure the attainment of plasma drug levels associated with the greatest likelihood of antidepressant response and the smallest risk of adverse effects.[191] TDM should be repeated when these drugs are being used to augment the effect of fluoxetine and paroxetine because of the substantial inhibition of CYP 2D6 caused by these two SSRIs (Table 6.11). When a TCA is added to a patient on fluoxetine, TDM of the TCA should be repeated every 1 to 2 weeks for at least 6 to 8 weeks. The reason for this recommendation is the long half-life of fluoxetine and its active metabolite, norfluoxetine. As their levels build, the functional activity of CYP 2D6 declines resulting in a gradual increase in the levels of the SATCAs.[186] The long half-life of norfluoxetine must also be considered when switching from fluoxetine to an SATCA or other drugs which are substrates of CYP enzymes moderately to substantially inhibited by norfluoxetine (Table

145

6.10). For a further discussion of this topic, refer to Chapter 10.

Disadvantages

Safety: While SATCAs avoid many of the actions which plague the use of TATCAs, they do inhibit Na^+ fast channels at only 10 times their usually effective concentrations.[194] For this reason, these antidepressants can be as lethal as the TATCAs following even a modest overdose.

Payment: Unlike the TATCAs, the cost of the generic versions of the SATCAs are not appreciably less than the newer antidepressants which do not have the same overdose lethality risk (Table 7.10).

Summary

The recommendation is to reserve SATCAs for refractory cases as either monodrug therapy or as a copharmacy strategy (Chapter 11).

When selecting an SATCA, some clinicians prefer nortriptyline because its optimal therapeutic plasma level range has been arguably better established. Others prefer desipramine because its adverse effect profile is arguably somewhat better.

Serotonin Selective Reuptake Inhibitors

This class of antidepressants has become the first choice for most prescribers (Table 8.1). SSRIs were the first class of antidepressant to be successfully developed using the approach of molecular targeting.[170] The goal was to produce antidepressants which both potently and selectively inhibited the serotonin uptake pump (Figure 6.1). That goal of selectivity was achieved for all members of this class in terms of neural mechanisms of action (Figure 6.3) but not in terms

146

of CYP enzymes (Figure 6.2). Figure 6.3 explains why members of this class are so similar in terms of their efficacy and adverse effect profile. Figure 6.2 explains why they are so different in terms of their risk of causing pharmacokinetic drug-drug interactions. The advantages and disadvantages of this class in general and specific members in particular are summarized below.

■ **Advantages**
- Good safety in the event of overdose due to a wide therapeutic index.
- Good safety in terms of pharmacodynamically mediated drug-drug interactions which are limited to those mediated by serotonin reuptake inhibition (eg, serotonin syndrome when combined with other serotonin agonists like MAOIs).[20,25,32,51,66,74,87,104,138,143,144,154,158,200,204,228,232,233]
- Good tolerability profile with virtually all of the adverse effects being consistent with excessive serotonin agonism:
  – Nausea
  – Loose stools
  – Sexual dysfunction (Table 6.6).
- Efficacy in outpatients with clinical depression which is comparable to any other type of antidepressant.[103]
- Efficacy in several anxiety disorders as well as clinical depression (Table 8.2).[103]
- Simplicity in terms of optimal dosing because of their flat dose-antidepressant response curve (ie, in fixed-dose clinical trials, there is not an average increase in response rate at doses above the usually effective, minimum dose). In the case of fluoxetine, paroxetine, and sertraline, the patient can be started at an effective dose without the need for titration. In the case of

TABLE 8.2 — INDICATIONS FORMALLY LABELED BY THE FDA FOR SPECIFIC SEROTONIN SELECTIVE REUPTAKE INHIBITORS*

SSRI	Depression	Obsessive-Compulsive Disorder	Panic Disorder	Bulimia Nervosa
Citalopram	Yes	No	No	No
Fluvoxamine	No	Yes	No	No
Fluoxetine	Yes	Yes	No	Yes
Paroxetine	Yes	Yes	Yes	No
Sertraline	Yes	Yes	Yes	No

Abbreviations: FDA, Food and Drug Administration; SSRI, serotonin selective reuptake inhibitor.

* All other antidepressants are solely labeled for the treatment of depression with the exception of bupropion which is marketed under the brand name Zyban as an aid for smoking cessation. Trials with venlafaxine are being reviewed by the FDA for possible labeling as indicated for the treatment of patients with generalized anxiety disorder. Trials with sertraline are being reviewed by the FDA for the possible labeling as indicated for the treatment of patients with double depression, dysthymia, and posttraumatic stress disorder.

citalopram and fluvoxamine, the recommended starting dose in their package insert was not found to be an effective dose in their clinical trials and thus an upward titration is recommended (Table 7.11). Also, all of the SSRIs (with the exception of fluvoxamine) are recommended to be taken once a day.

■ Disadvantages

Disadvantages of SSRIs can be broken down into two types:
- Those shared by the SSRIs as a group
- Those which are limited to only certain SSRIs.

Although SSRIs have a good tolerability profile, their adverse effects can be rate-limiting for some patients. That is particularly true for the sexual dysfunction caused by these drugs.[145,147] Some patients will discontinue SSRIs during the maintenance phase because of this adverse effect, putting themselves at risk for a recurrent episode. Approaches that have been tried to minimize this adverse effect are further discussed in Chapter 11.

Like any antidepressant class, SSRIs do not treat all patients with clinical depression. They produce a full remission in approximately 50% of patients. Although it is a popular strategy to try a second SSRI in a patient who has not benefited from a trial of a first SSRI, there is no compelling scientific data to support this practice (Chapter 11). Moreover, the pharmacology of these drugs suggest that this strategy should only work in those patients who do not develop adequate plasma levels of the first SSRI.[170] Since the SSRIs do not share the same pharmacokinetics (ie, metabolic pathways) (Table 6.9), there is a percentage of the population who will respond to a second SSRI, but the percentage is likely to be small. A switch to a different mechanism of action or an augmentation strategy would seem the more prudent course of action in such cases (Chapter 11).

As discussed in Chapter 6, a serotonin withdrawal syndrome (Table 6.13) can occur following the discontinuation of any SSRI. However, the likelihood and the severity is inversely related to the half-life of the SSRI, being most common on fluvoxamine and paroxetine, less on citalopram and sertraline, and the least on fluoxetine. Generally, this problem can be avoided or minimized by slowly tapering fluvoxamine or paroxetine. When this tactic does not work, the patient can be switched to fluoxetine, which can then be stopped in this manner. This strategy is analogous to using clonazepam to taper patients off of alprazolam (ie, using a long-lived drug to taper patients of a short-lived drug with the same pharmacodynamics).

While the above disadvantages are shared by all SSRIs, there are others which are not. The most important of these non-shared disadvantages is the fact that three SSRIs inhibit one or more drug-metabolizing CYP enzyme(s) to a substantial degree and thus have the potential for causing clinically important pharmacokinetic drug-drug interactions (Figure 6.2 and Table 6.10). These three SSRIs are:

- Fluoxetine *Prozac*
- Fluvoxamine *Luvox*
- Paroxetine. *Paxil*

Substantial inhibition means coadministration of these SSRIs causes a several-fold increase in the levels of the coprescribed "victim" drugs which are dependent on the inhibited CYP enzyme for their clearance. The increased accumulation of the "victim" drug can result in dose-dependent adverse effects that present in a myriad of ways. Given the importance of this topic for medicine in general, it is further discussed in Chapter 10 with case examples of how such drug-drug interactions can present clinically. Briefly, this issue is important for multiple reasons:

- The majority of patients taking an antidepressant are likely to be also on at least one other systemically taken, prescription medication in addition to their antidepressant. Such patients are at risk for a drug-drug interaction.
- Cytochrome P450 enzyme-mediated drug-drug interactions are the most common types of clinically important pharmacokinetic drug-drug interactions.
- The consequence of such interactions may be erroneously attributed to either a sensitivity problem on the part of the patient or even to a worsening of the patient's underlying health problems.
- The inhibition of CYP enzymes conveys no known therapeutic advantage to outweigh the problems posed.

This difference among SSRIs stems from the fact that when they were developed, drug-development scientists were not able to screen for effects on CYP enzymes which mediate the bulk of oxidative drug metabolism.[223] That is unfortunate because these effects on CYP enzymes unnecessarily complicate the use of fluoxetine, fluvoxamine, and paroxetine in the patient on other medications.

Given these facts, it is somewhat surprising that fluoxetine and paroxetine are still prescribed as frequently as they are (Table 8.1). That is particularly true for fluoxetine since it inhibits multiple CYP enzymes and this inhibition can persist for weeks after it has been discontinued due to the long half-life of the parent drug and its active metabolite, norfluoxetine.[186] Clinicians need to be mindful of this issue when prescribing another drug to a patient who has been on fluoxetine, even weeks after it has been stopped.

Fortunately, the practitioner has two SSRI options which do not carry substantial liability in terms of CYP enzyme inhibition:

- Citalopram *Celexa*
- Sertraline. *Zoloft*

These two SSRIs have all the advantages of this class without the disadvantage of CYP enzyme inhibition (Figure 6.2 and Table 6.10).

■ Summary

The SSRIs for many clinicians have become the treatment of first choice for the majoritiy of their patients with clinical depression due to their safety, tolerability and simplicity when used alone (Table 8.1). All of the members of this class share these advantages.

Members of this class differ substantially with regard to their safety, tolerability and simplicity when used in a patient on other medications (Chapter 10). Three of the SSRIs (fluoxetine, fluvoxamine and paroxetine) produce substantial inhibition of drug metabolizing CYP enzymes.

While citalopram and sertraline share many of the same advantages over the other SSRIs, sertraline:

- Has been much more extensively studied in terms of drug-drug interactions[172,223]
- Has Food and Drug Administration (FDA)-approved indications for anxiety disorders in addition to major depression, specifically:
  - Panic disorder
  - Obsessive-compulsive disorder (Table 8.2)[273]
- Has a recommended starting dose which is usually effective (Table 7.11).

Serotonin and Norepinephrine Reuptake Inhibitors

Venlafaxine is the only member of this class available in the United States (Table 6.2). Several other drugs in this class are or have been in clinical trials in the United States and other countries. Venlafaxine has dose-dependent, sequential effects on the uptake pumps for serotonin and then norepinephrine (Figure 6.4). At 75 mg/day, venlafaxine is predominantly a serotonin reuptake inhibitor (SRI) like the SSRIs. At 375 mg/day, it produces comparable norepinephrine uptake inhibition to an NSRI such as desipramine. This pharmacology is consistent with the advantages and disadvantages of this antidepressant.

■ **Advantages**
- Good safety in the event of overdose due to a wide therapeutic index.[73,103]
- Good safety in terms of pharmacodynamically mediated drug-drug interactions. At lower doses, these are limited to those mediated by serotonin reuptake inhibition (eg, serotonin syndrome when combined with other serotonin agonists like MAOIs). At higher doses, it is also susceptible to the same potential interactions as an NSRI (eg, hypertensive crisis when combined with other norepinephrine agonists, particularly MAOIs).[73,151]
- Good safety in terms of pharmacokinetically mediated drug-drug interactions. Like citalopram and sertraline—but in contrast to fluoxetine, fluvoxamine, nefazodone, and paroxetine—venlafaxine does not produce substantial inhibition of any drug metabolizing CYP enzyme at its usually effective, minimum antidepressant dose (Table 6.10).

- Good tolerability profile. At low doses, its adverse effects profile is similar to that of an SSRI:
  - Nausea
  - Loose stools
  - Sexual dysfunction (Tables 6.5 and 6.7).
- At higher doses, it can also produce the same adverse effects as an NSRI:
  - Mild increase in blood pressure
  - Increased diaphoresis
  - Tachycardia
  - Tremors
  - Anxiety (Tables 6.5 and 6.7).[151,171]
- Efficacy at 75 mg/day is comparable to any other type of antidepressant in outpatients with clinical depression.[169]
- Better efficacy at higher doses. Venlafaxine has an ascending dose-response curve in terms of antidepressant efficacy in contrast to the SSRIs. That is consistent with its sequential effects on serotonin and norepinephrine uptake inhibition (Figure 6.4 and Table 6.2). In essence, a dose increase with venlafaxine is pharmacologically and clinically a built-in augmentation strategy comparable to adding an NSRI such as desipramine to an SSRI such as sertraline.[177] At doses of 225 mg/day, venlafaxine was superior to 40 mg/day of fluoxetine in treating hospitalized patients with clinical depression.[48] In another study, a dose increase of venlafaxine converted more nonresponders to responders than did a comparable dose increase of fluoxetine.[52]
- Simplicity in terms of optimal dosing because of the ability to prescribe a usually effective dose (ie, 75 mg/day) from the beginning without the need for dose titration. As a result of

the development of the extended release version, venlafaxine can be taken once a day.

■ Disadvantages

- A somewhat higher incidence of gastrointestinal adverse effects compared to SSRIs (Table 6.7 versus Table 6.5). In particular, nausea appears to be more common when taking venlafaxine than most of the SSRIs.
- Has the same liability for causing sexual dysfunction as the SSRIs.[103]
- Has adrenergically mediated adverse effects at higher doses.[151,171]
- Due to its relatively short half-life, venlafaxine has a risk of causing the serotonin withdrawal syndrome (Table 6.13) comparable to that of fluvoxamine and paroxetine.[219] The incidence and the severity of the serotonin withdrawal syndrome is in part a function of the half-life of the SRI. The half-life of venlafaxine, including that of its active metabolite O-desmethylvenlafaxine, is approximately 12 hours.[119] The extended-release formulation of venlafaxine does not change the half-life of venlafaxine and thus does not change the risk of the serotonin withdrawal syndrome following abrupt venlafaxine discontinuation. While this withdrawal state is not as medically serious as the sedative-hypnotic withdrawal syndrome, it is not innocuous and can be quite unpleasant. Some patients may mistake the withdrawal symptoms for a relapse of their depressive illness and can become so dysphoric or agitated that they can experience suicidal ideations.[209,210] It can also mimic mania which may lead to a misdiagnosis and inappropriate treatment.[125]
- Ironically, dosing with venlafaxine can be viewed as either an advantage or a disadvan-

155

tage. It is an advantage in that the patient can be started on an effective dose (as with SSRIs) at the beginning of treatment. Moreover, there is more compelling evidence to try a higher dose of venlafaxine in a patient who has not benefited from the usual starting dose than is the case with the SSRIs. Nevertheless, the ability to titrate the dose of venlafaxine means that the practitioner may feel less certain about what constitutes an optimal trial of this antidepressant.

■ **Summary**

Venlafaxine is a dual action drug that predominantly acts like an SSRI at low doses and adds the effect of an NSRI at high doses (Table 6.2 and Figure 6.1). Like citalopram and sertraline and in contrast to fluoxetine, fluvoxamine, nefazodone, and paroxetine, it has minimal effects on CYP enzymes (Table 6.10).

Serotonin 2A Receptor Blockade and Weak Serotonin Reuptake Inhibition

This class includes both nefazodone and its precursor, trazodone. More prescriptions are written for trazodone than nefazodone (Table 8.1), most likely reflecting the extensive use of trazodone as a nonhabit-forming sleep aid rather than as an antidepressant. Nefazodone is a structural analogue of trazodone and was designed with the goal of producing a better antidepressant than trazodone.[271] Specifically, nefazodone is a less potent antihistamine than trazodone. The antihistaminergic properties of trazodone are in part responsible for its popularity as a sleep aid, but cause significant problems with daytime sedation when it is used as an antidepressant. Nefazodone is also a more potent SRI than trazodone. Nevertheless, nefazodone is a much weaker SRI than the SSRIs and venlafaxine.[31,77] Nefazodone likely only produces serotonin (5-HT)-2A inhibition at doses ≤ 300 mg/day and even at doses of 500 mg/day does not appear to produce the same degree of the serotonin reuptake inhibition as occurs with the SSRIs and venlafaxine at their starting doses.[150] This pharmacology is consistent with the clinical advantages and disadvantages of nefazodone.

■ **Advantages**
- Good safety in overdose due to a wide therapeutic index.[208]
- It does not disturb sleep physiology and improves the subjective quality of sleep.[10,82]
- It appears to cause minimal sexual dysfunction.[103]
- Efficacy in patients with clinical depression and prominent anxiety.[71]

■ **Disadvantages**
- Risk of pharmacokinetically mediated drug-drug interactions. Due to the inhibition of the drug metabolizing CYP 3A3/4 enzyme, nefazodone has the potential to cause CYP enzyme-mediated drug-drug interactions like fluoxetine, fluvoxamine, and paroxetine (Table 6.10). Nefazodone-induced inhibition of CYP 3A3/4 can elevate levels of coprescribed drugs dependent on this CYP enzyme for their oxidative metabolism (Table 6.9) and that, in turn, can cause untoward consequences.[223]
- Tolerability problems limit the starting dose of nefazodone.[171] The incidence and severity of the following adverse effects increase as a function of the starting dose of nefazodone:
  – Dizziness/lightheadedness

8

- Confusion
- Sedation
- Gastrointestinal adverse effects (Table 6.7). Stepwise dose titration allows the patient to develop some tolerance for these effects. The package insert advises starting nefazodone at 100 mg twice a day for 1 week before increasing in increments of 100 to 200 mg/day at intervals no less than 1 week (Table 7.11). Using this strategy, the dose of nefazodone can be increased as needed to a maximum of 600 mg/day in equally divided doses administered 2 or 3 times per day. Such a titration schedule means more clinician time, more patient education, and more chances that the patient will call back with issues or questions.

- Antidepressant efficacy at its initial starting dose is less robust than with other antidepressants.[103,177] There is no compelling evidence that nefazodone has antidepressant efficacy at a dose of 200 mg/day. In fact, doses of 400 to 500 mg/day are required to produce the same degree of antidepressant efficacy as the SSRIs and venlafaxine at their starting doses as measured by the drop in the Hamilton Depression Rating Scale scores in clinical trials.[103,177] That suggests that blockade of the 5-HT2A alone is not a robust mechanism for antidepressant efficacy (Table 6.2). As the dose of nefazodone increases, serotonin reuptake inhibition is added to its overall effect. Thus, dose titration is needed when prescribing nefazodone both to improve its tolerability and increase its antidepressant efficacy.

- Simplicity of dosing and difficulty establishing the optimal dose. While the tolerability and efficacy issues described above account for much of the problem in dosing nefazodone, its pharmacokinetics, including its effects on the drug metabolizing CYP 3A, are also important as follows:

– Nefazodone has nonlinear pharmacokinetics (ie, its plasma levels increase disproportionately to dose increases).[109] A four-fold increase in dose can produce a 14-fold increase in the plasma concentrations of the parent drug.

– Nefazodone at low doses has low bioavailability (ie, approximately 20% of the dose reaches the systemic circulation) due to high first pass metabolism via the CYP 3A enzyme.[103]

– Since nefazodone inhibits CYP 3A, it inhibits its own first pass metabolism. For that reason, its bioavailability (ie, the fraction of the dose reaching the systemic circulation) increases as its dose increases. Since the acute adverse effects of nefazodone (as with many drugs) are dose dependent, its nonlinear pharmacokinetics contribute to the higher frequency and severity of adverse effects at higher starting doses.

• The metabolism of nefazodone is also complicated in that the parent drug has a relatively short half-life of approximately 4 hours and is converted into three pharmacologically active metabolites:

– Hydroxynefazodone
– Triazoledione
– Meta-chlorophenylpiperazine (mCPP).[139]

Hydroxynefazodone has the same *in vitro* pharmacology as the parent drug and, thus, is believed to have the same clinical pharmacology.[237] The *in vitro* pharmacology of the other two metabolites differs substantially from that of the parent drug. The triazoledione metabolite is a relatively pure 5-HT2A antagonist and hence its contribution to the antidepressant activity of nefazodone is uncertain.[237] The mCPP metabolite is a 5-HT2C agonist and, when given alone, causes anxiety and restlessness.[42,107] Unusually high accumulation of this metabolite occurs in approximately 7% of Caucasians because its clearance is dependent on the genetically polymorphic CYP 2D6 enzyme.

- The role of CYP 2D6 in the clearance of mCPP takes on additional significance if the patient is being switched from fluoxetine or paroxetine to nefazodone because these two SSRIs substantially inhibit this drug metabolizing CYP enzyme at their usually effective antidepressant dose (Table 6.11). In fact, fluoxetine at a dose of 20 mg/day has been shown to produce approximately an 800% increase in mCPP levels (Table 6.11). Although not formally studied, paroxetine at 20 mg/day would be expected to produce comparable increases in mCPP levels based on studies with other CYP 2D6 substrates (Table 6.11). This action on CYP 2D6-mediated metabolism of mCPP likely accounts for the paradoxical reactions that can occur when switching patients from either fluoxetine or paroxetine to nefazodone.

- Nefazodone typically improves sleep and decreases anxiety; yet, mCPP given alone does the opposite.[42,107] In most patients, mCPP levels are not sufficiently high to offset the effects of the parent drug, but these levels can be high enough in patients who are either genetically deficient in CYP 2D6 or who have been made functionally deficient in CYP 2D6 as a result of treatment with either fluoxetine or paroxetine (Table 6.11). The greater accumulation of this metabolite leads to greater 5-HT2C agonism which can in turn interact pharmacodynamically with persistent serotonin reuptake inhibition produced by fluoxetine's long-lived active metabolite, norfluoxetine.[197]

■ Summary

All of the above factors cause an apparently greater degree of interpatient variability in terms of response to nefazodone than is true for many of the other new antidepressants. Nevertheless, nefazodone can be a useful antidepressant option for the primary-care practitioner for selected patients such as those who do not tolerate the adverse effects caused by serotonin reuptake inhibition.

Specific Serotonin and Adrenergic Receptor Blockers

Mirtazapine is the only member of this class available in the United States, although its predecessor, mianserin, is available in other countries. The mechanism of action of mirtazapine is unique.[58,59,77] It does not block the uptake pump for any of the biogenic amine neurotransmitters (ie, serotonin, norepinephrine, and dopamine). Instead, mirtazapine blocks histamine-1 receptors (its most potent action) and specific serotonin and adrenergic receptors: the 5-HT2A, 5-HT2C, 5-HT3 and alpha-2–adrenergic receptors (Figure 6.4).[58,59,77] These actions are believed to mediate its antidepressant activity by increasing the release of serotonin and norepinephrine and hence their availability to their respective synaptic receptors. The blockade of the 5-HT2A, 5-HT2C, and 5-HT3 receptors is postulated to result in a selective increase in serotonin availability to the 5-HT1A receptor which has been implicated in the pathophysiology of clinical depression. Regardless of whether this postulated mechanism is correct, mirtazapine has been shown in clinical trials to have antidepressant activity. The pharmacology of mirtazapine is consistent with its beneficial and adverse effects.

■ Advantages
- Good safety in overdose.[33,151]
- Probably good safety in terms of pharmacokinetically mediated drug-drug interactions based on *in vitro* studies which show minimal potency for inhibiting any of the major drug-metabolizing CYP enzymes.[178] However, this *in vitro* prediction should be tested by appropriate *in vivo* studies.

- Mirtazapine does not cause many of the adverse effects seen with SRIs (Tables 6.5 and 6.7). Specifically, it does not:
  - Cause nausea or loose stools
  - Disturb sleep physiology (actually, it increases sleep efficiency, most likely as a result of its blockade of both histamine-1 and 5-HT2A receptors)[77]
  - Cause sexual dysfunction.
- Efficacy in patients with prominent anxiety consistent with the fact that mirtazapine blocks the 5-HT2A and 5-HT2C receptors.[267]
- Efficacy in severely depressed patients. Mirtazapine was found to be superior to fluoxetine in the treatment of hospitalized patients with clinical depression in one double-blind random assignment clinical trial.[267]
- Simplicity of dosing. Mirtazapine can be started on a dose which is effective in treating clinical depression and is taken once a day.

■ Disadvantages
- Safety: There were three cases of agranulocytosis out of 3000 patients in its clinical trial program.[151,178] That incidence was too low to draw

a cause and effect conclusion. Postmarketing experience with the drug has not inidicated an unusual number of cases of agranulocytosis in patients on this antidepressant. Nevertheless, the package insert contains a warning that a white blood cell count should be done if a patient on mirtazapine develops signs of fever or infection.

- Tolerability: Consistent with its histamine-1 receptor blockade, mirtazapine is sedating, which can be helpful for the patient with prominent insomnia, but can persist well into the next day consistent with its half-life. Sedation was listed as the reason for early termination in 10% of patients in its double-blind registration studies.[203] Although it may initially seem paradoxical, higher doses of mirtazapine theoretically could decrease its sedative effects. The postulated explanation is that mirtazapine's most potent action is histamine-1 receptor blockade, but at higher levels, mirtazapine also blocks the alpha-2–adrenergic receptor (Figure 6.4). That latter action causes an alerting effect which could counteract the sedation produced by the more potent effect, central histamine blockade (Figure 6.4).

- Consistent with its 5-HT2C blockade, mirtazapine can cause an increase in appetite and weight gain (Table 6.7). These effects can be desirable in specific patients (eg, patients with clinical depression and a concomitant medical problem such as cancer which causes failure to thrive). However, these effects were also listed as the reason for early termination in 8% of patients in the mirtazapine registration studies.[203]

- Difficulty establishing the optimal dose. Appropriate double-blind, fixed-dose studies have not been published with mirtazapine. Therefore, the optimal dose has not been established. There is also no rigorous information on what is the appropriate course of action if the patient does not respond to the initial dose.

■ **Summary**

Mirtazapine may never achieve the level of use of some of the other newer antidepressants (Table 8.1). Nevertheless, its unique pharmacology make it a useful antidepressant option for selected patients.

Dopamine and Norepinephrine Reuptake Inhibitors

Bupropion is the only drug in this class labeled for the treatment of clinical depression. However, psychostimulants (eg, methylphenidate) share its pharmacological actions on the dopamine and norepinephrine uptake pumps.

■ **Advantages**
- Better safety in overdose than tricyclic antidepressants, but can cause seizures.[57]
- Risk of pharmacodynamically mediated drug-drug interactions comparable to that of the NSRIs.
- Tolerability profile comparable to an NSRI and distinct from that of an SSRI (Table 6.7 versus Table 6.5). Specifically, bupropion does not disturb sleep physiology. It causes minimal, if any, sexual dysfunction.[213] In fact, some practitioners have reported success in using bupropion as an add-on to treat SSRI-induced sexual dysfunction (Chapter 11).

- Efficacy: Consistent with its dopamine and norepinephrine uptake inhibition, bupropion is an activating antidepressant and could be particularly useful in patients with prominent psychomotor retardation (Tables 6.5 and 6.7). Given its dopamine agonistic properties, it could also be uniquely helpful in the patient with Parkinson's disease as well as in patients with attention deficit/hyperactivity disorder.[265] Theoretically, bupropion may work in patients who have not benefited from a trial of an SRI since bupropion inhibits norepinephrine as well as dopamine uptake (Table 6.2 and Figure 6.4).[30] Recall that NSRIs such as desipramine have been found to work in 50% of patients who do not benefit from SSRIs.[245] Nevertheless, no formal studies have been done with bupropion to test this possibility.

- Efficacy: Bupropion has also gained FDA approval as an aid in smoking cessation.[274] That is relevant to its use as an antidepressant because smokers have an increased incidence of clinical depression in comparison to nonsmokers and clinical depression impairs the ability to stop smoking. Thus, bupropion could serve a dual role—both to treat the clinical depression and as an aid to stop smoking.

■ Disadvantages

- Safety: This antidepressant has a narrow therapeutic index in terms of the dose needed for antidepressant efficacy versus the dose that causes seizures.[57] The minimum recommended dose for antidepressant response is 300 mg/day and a number of patients will need the maximum recommended dose of 450 mg/day. At doses of 450 mg/day or less, the seizure risk is 0.4%. Doubling the dose to 900 mg/day causes a five-fold increase in the seizure risk.[57] Given the dose-dependent nature of the seizures, patients who seize on lower doses are probably slow metabolizers who accumulate unusually high levels of bupropion or its three active metabolites.[180] For that reason, TDM is a potential way to further minimize this risk, but TDM with bupropion has not been adequately studied.[180] Particular care should be taken when switching from an antidepressant, which substantially inhibits specific drug-metabolizing CYP enzymes (ie, fluoxetine, fluvoxamine, nefazodone, or paroxetine), to bupropion, or when adding bupropion to the treatment regimen of patients on these antidepressants or on other drugs which substantially inhibit CYP enzymes (eg, macrolides, fluoroquinoles, antifungals, protease inhibitors).

- Uncertainty about its potential to cause pharmacokinetically mediated drug-drug interactions. Bupropion is one of the oldest of the new antidepressants.[196] The clinical trials that originally led to its registration were conducted in the middle to the late 1970s. For that reason, little has been done to formally test the potential effects of bupropion on CYP enzymes. There have been case reports that coadministration of bupropion can substantially affect the metabolism of the TATCA, imipramine.[225] This finding suggests that bupropion or one of its metabolites inhibits CYP 2D6, but that possibility has not been formally tested. Conversely, there are also case reports that coadministration of fluoxetine can substantially increase the plasma levels of two of the metabolites of bupropion.[180] Again, the CYP enzyme mediating this effect has not been established, but raises the possibility that bupropion could be the target as well as the cause of CYP enzyme-mediated pharmacokinetic drug-drug interactions. That is potentially important due to the dose and hence concentration-dependent nature of the risk of seizures in patients on bupropion.[57]

- Simplicity of dosing: The recommended dosing guidelines with the immediate-release version of bupropion is for 3 times a day administration. Doses should not be administered closer than 4 hours apart.[57] This schedule was based on the half-life of bupropion and the concern about its seizure risk being related to peak levels of bupropion and/or its metabolites. A sustained-release version of bupropion has been marketed. Unfortunately, this formulation did not achieve the goal of once-a-day dosing. Instead, the recommendation is to give the sustained-release formulation twice a day. Even with this sustained-release version, there is still the recommendation that the dose should not be taken closer than 4 hours apart.

- Difficulty establishing the optimal dose. The optimal dose of bupropion has not been established using fixed-dose trials. When prescribing this antidepressant, the goal is to keep the dose as low as possible to minimize the risk of seizures without compromising therapeutic efficacy.

■ Summary

The seizure risk with bupropion, while not as serious as the cardiotoxicity of the TCAs, initially limited its use. Its clinical acceptance has been helped by its labeling as an aid in smoking cessation and by the development of a sustained-release formulation (Table 8.1). Bupropion is a useful option for patients who do not benefit from or tolerate SRIs. It may be the best choice for the patient with comorbid Parkinson's disease since its mechanism of action could potentiate the beneficial effects of L-dopa.[195] Certainly, bupropion should not aggravate Parkinson's disease as can happen with SRIs because the serotonin is an inhibitory afferent into the dopamine neurons in the substantia nigra.[111,174] Given its pharmacological similarities to methylphenidate, bupropion might also be uniquely effective in patients with both residual attention deficit symptoms and clinical depression.

Monoamine Oxidase Inhibitors

These antidepressants are rarely used by psychiatrists, and even less by other clinicians. Nevertheless, they deserve some comments for the sake of completeness.

■ Advantages

These antidepressants can be used effectively and safely assuming the prescriber is knowledgeable with regard to proper patient selection and education, and is conscientious with regard to monitoring the course of treatment. They can work in patients whose depressive illness is refractory to other forms of antidepressant pharmacology. For these reasons, they remain valuable antidepressant options.[243]

■ Disadvantages

Potentially fatal pharmacodynamic drug-drug interactions can occur with MAOIs when combined with a variety of drugs which are serotonin agonists (ie, the serotonin syndrome), norepinephrine agonists, or with foods rich in tyramine (ie, hypertensive crisis).[103] The major adverse effect that occurs on MAOIs alone is hypotension which can present as fatigue and may mimic worsening of the underlying depressive syndrome. For this reason, the blood pressure should be monitored when using these antidepressants.[103]

168

■ Summary

For patients who need them, the benefits of the MAOIs can outweigh their liabilities.

Summary

This chapter provides a framework for understanding the clinical pharmacology of the various antidepressants and presents the available clinical data in a way that should aid in optimally selecting an antidepressant for a specific patient. The relative advantages and disadvantages are given for the various classes of antidepressants and within classes for individual members when appropriate. Given the pharmacological differences between the various classes of antidepressant, the choice of a specific medication for a specific patient will often be dependent on the symptom cluster.

Another basis for choosing a specific antidepressant is when a patient has not benefited from an earlier trial with an antidepressant (Chapter 11). Faced with this situation, many practitioners chose to try another antidepressant from the same class, particularly in terms of trying a second or even a third SSRI. Given the unfortunate lack of data, the wisdom of this approach is debatable. Based on pharmacology, it would seem more prudent to switch to a class with a different mechanism of action than to stay within the same class (Table 6.2 and Chapter 11).

Finally, there are sufficient differences among the antidepressants that the final decision may come down to personal preference. For example, does the clinician prefer the advantages of a single-mechanism-of-action antidepressant or a dual-mechanism-of-action drug? The former simplifies dosing and the adverse effect profile, but has potential limitations in terms of antidepressant response. Should the patient not benefit from treatment with an antidepressant having a

8

single mechanism of action, dose escalation is less likely to be a useful way of increasing efficacy. In such instances, the practitioner could either switch to an antidepressant with a different mechanism of action or use an augmentation strategy by adding a drug with another mechanism of action (Chapter 11).

In the case of the antidepressant with dual mechanisms of action, the augmentation strategy may be built-in and the approach would be to escalate the dose. However, that means the determination of the optimal dose is more of an issue than is true for an antidepressant with a single mechanism of action. Moreover, multiple mechanisms can contribute to more adverse effects and increase the potential for pharmacodynamic drug-drug interactions. For all of these reasons, the issue of choosing between a single versus a dual mechanism of action antidepressant becomes a matter of personal preference and clinical experience.

9

What to Do After the Medication Has Been Selected

Treatment begins with the selection of an antidepressant for the patient. This chapter will review the process to optimally manage the patient after treatment has begun, including:

- Monitoring the initial phase of treatment to ensure that optimal response is achieved
- Educating the patient about the drug treatment so the patient will know what to expect
- Informing the patient about the nature of the illness and the patient's role in treatment to achieve an optimal recovery from the illness. That education must include a discussion of the fact that in many cases clinical depression is a episodic, recurrent illness.

The goal is to have the patient be an active and important part of the treatment team to increase the likelihood of the optimal recovery from the illness.

Initiation and Follow-Up of an Antidepressant Trial

Optimal treatment starts with appropriate patient education about the nature of the illness and the nature of the proposed treatment. That discussion should include:

- The reasons for selecting a specific medication
- When to expect improvement in depressive symptoms

- How that improvement is likely to manifest itself
- What adverse effects the patient may experience
- What to do in the event adverse effects occur.

A script for patient education has been provided in Chapter 4.

The goal of such education is to help the patient be an active participant in his/her treatment. That, in turn, should enhance compliance. The rationale is that patients are more likely to remain on a treatment even if it causes a nuisance adverse effect when they know what to expect and what to do if it occurs. They are also more likely to inform the clinician if they experience an unexpected effect, thus diminishing the likelihood of a serious adverse outcome.

The appropriate interval between the initial visit and the first follow-up visit will typically be either 1 or 2 weeks depending on how well the patient will likely tolerate the medication. The patient should be instructed to either call the clinic or decrease the dose if s/he is having any adverse effects that are more than a nuisance. At the return visit, the practitioner can assess the adequacy of the dosing schedule, determine how well the medication is working, and in the case of a tricyclic antidepressant (TCA), obtain a plasma sample to measure the plasma drug level to guide further dose adjustment (Figure 9.1).[191]

As discussed in Chapter 8, some antidepressants can cause adverse effects which can be treatment limiting even though not medically serious. In such instances, a closer follow-up may be useful to assess the patient's response, provide reassurance, and take any corrective steps that may be needed (Chapter 11). An example would be the sedative action of mirtazapine which occurs early in treatment, often after the first dose.[151,178] While this sedation is usually not medically serious, it can lead to patient discontinuation. The clinician may choose to deal with that issue by phone if it arises or may wish to schedule a closer follow-up visit to assess the situation.

During interval visits, patient education about the illness and its treatment should continue by:

- Responding to any patient questions
- Clarifying issues as needed
- Providing support and encouragement by addressing any intervening issues (eg, family or employment stresses)
- Assessing the safety, tolerability, and efficacy of the medication trial.

Obviously, the more severe the episode, the closer the follow-up should be. Given the fact that all of the current classes of antidepressants have a delayed onset of clinically significant antidepressant activity, the clinician may want to see the markedly ill patient sooner if there is a possibility that suicidal ideation may emerge between starting the medication and substantial improvement in the depressive episode.

The interval between follow-up is also dependent on whether the practitioner needs to see the patient to:

- Assess response
- Titrate the dose
- Deal with the likelihood of treatment-limiting adverse effects.

The variables that will go into that decision include:

- The personal preferences of the practitioner
- The nature of the patient, including the nature of the depressive illness
- The specific medication selected.

Even a one- or two-step dose titration schedule can be accomplished without requiring an early return visit. It does require active patient participation and hence proper patient education. For example, a patient who is going to be treated with desipramine can be instructed to start with 50 mg/day for 3 days, advance to 75 mg/day for 3 days, and then to 100 mg/day until s/he returns to see the clinician.

The patient with a first-time episode of clinical depression has a 50:50 chance of having another episode some time in the future.[4,61,98] The likelihood increases if the patient has a strong positive family history for recurrent depressive illness. The patient should be educated about the early warning signs of a recurrent episode to reduce the time between when the patient experiences the onset of an episode and when s/he seeks help. That, in turn, hopefully will reduce the severity and the duration of the episode.

It is useful to explain to the patient with a single depressive episode that there is a good chance s/he will not have another one. In the event another episode occurs, there may be years between the episodes. It should also be emphasized that should future episodes occur, they should be just as responsive to medication as the first one was. There is no reason why the patient should not have a full, productive, and happy life. The goal is to provide a realistic recognition that there is a chance of a recurrence without overemphasizing the risk and producing the depressive equivalent of a "cardiac cripple."

At the end of a 4- to 6-week trial of the medication, the patient's response can be assessed (Figure 9.1). The response can be divided into three categories:

- Full remission
- Partial response
- No response.

These categories have been defined in Table 5.1. There are several rating scales that have been developed to provide a reliable quantification of the severity of the patient's depressive episode and response

174

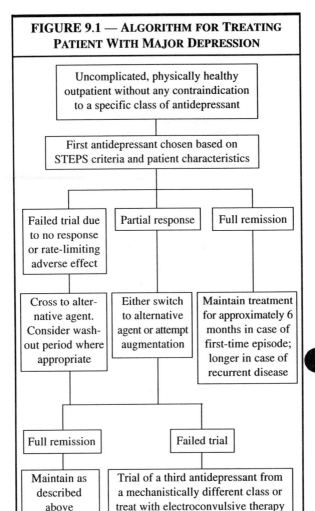

FIGURE 9.1 — ALGORITHM FOR TREATING PATIENT WITH MAJOR DEPRESSION

Uncomplicated, physically healthy outpatient without any contraindication to a specific class of antidepressant

First antidepressant chosen based on STEPS criteria and patient characteristics

Failed trial due to no response or rate-limiting adverse effect

Partial response

Full remission

Cross to alternative agent. Consider washout period where appropriate

Either switch to alternative agent or attempt augmentation

Maintain treatment for approximately 6 months in case of first-time episode; longer in case of recurrent disease

Full remission

Failed trial

Maintain as described above

Trial of a third antidepressant from a mechanistically different class or treat with electroconvulsive therapy

9

FIGURE 9.2 — ZUNG DEPRESSION SELF-REPORT RATING SCALE

Name _____

Age _____ Sex _____ Date _____

Please put a check in the box that best reflects how you have mainly felt in the past week for each question.

	None	Some	Mostly	Always
1. I feel downhearted, blue, and sad				
2. Morning is when I feel the best				
3. I have crying spells or feel like it				
4. I have trouble sleeping through the night				
5. I eat as much as I used to				
6. I enjoy looking at, talking to, and being with attractive women/men				
7. I notice that I am losing weight				
8. I have trouble with constipation				
9. My heart beats faster than usual				
10. I get tired for no reason				
11. My mind is as clear as it used to be				
12. I find it easy to do the things I used to do				
13. I am restless and can't keep still				
14. I feel hopeful about the future				
15. I am more irritable than usual				

	None	Some	Mostly	Always
16. I find it easy to make decisions				
17. I feel that I am useful and needed				
18. My life is pretty full				
19. I feel that others would be better off if I were dead				
20. I still enjoy the things I used to do				

to treatment. The one that is most readily adapted to the primary-care setting is the patient self-report questionnaire, the Zung Depression Self-Report Rating Scale (Figure 9.2). This form can be given to the patient to complete before the clinician sees the patient. This approach increases efficiency and reinforces patient education. By completing this form, the patient learns to think about the severity of his/her illness in a more precise and quantifiable way. This education can facilitate the patient's ability to monitor his/her progress.

9

Duration of Continuation Therapy

If this is a first episode, the patient should remain on the antidepressant for at least 4 months after remission.[4,61,98] This interval is a vulnerable period during which the probability of a relapse is high if the patient does not remain on medication.

During this phase, the patient should be seen generally every 1 to 2 months for follow-up medication checks. During these visits, the practitioner will determine whether the medication continues to be effective in terms of maintaining remission and whether it continues to be well-tolerated and safe. In addition, education about the illness continues by clarifying any questions that the patient may have. This education includes a reiteration of the rationale for maintenance therapy: its purpose and its projected duration.

At the last few visits prior to the termination of continuation therapy, education should shift to the likelihood of a recurrent episode. This training can help the patient be more sensitive to the recurrence of symptoms after the antidepressant medication has been stopped as discussed below.

Maintenance Therapy

Antidepressant medication can be used to prevent future episodes as well as to treat current ones. If the patient has had two previous episodes, there is almost a 90% chance of having future episodes after medication is discontinued.[4,61,98] Even so, the next episode may be years into the future (ie, every 10 years). Indefinite therapy for all such patients seems excessive. Instead, each episode may be treated separately. For patients with seasonal onset to their depressive illness, they may discontinue the medication during the seasons when they are not at risk for a recurrence, but initiate therapy shortly before entering the season at risk.[103]

Clearly, there are some patients for whom the benefits of indefinite antidepressant treatment outweigh the downside. Ideally, the patient should make this decision based on balancing the following factors: the frequency, severity, duration, and recurrent depressive episodes versus problems or inconveniences associated with maintenance antidepressant therapy. Follow-up visits during active prophylactic treatment may be a number of months apart, depending on how long the patient has been on the antidepressant and the nature of his/her depressive illness.

10 Use of Antidepressants With Other Medications

The preceding chapters have focused on the antidepressant alone; however, the majority of patients on an antidepressant seen in primary-care settings are on other medications as well (Table 10.1). In this chapter, the potential downside of polydrug therapy will be discussed as a cautionary note. In the next chapter, the upside of polydrug therapy will be discussed; specifically, from the perspective of adding other drugs to either treat tolerability problems or augment antidepressant efficacy.

This chapter then will focus on the caution that should be exercised when using polydrug therapy. It will discuss the potential for adverse outcome resulting from an unintended drug-drug interaction.

To understand the potential magnitude of this problem, consider the percentage of patients on an antidepressant in different practice settings who are on more than one other medication and thus at risk for having a drug-drug interaction. In both primary-care and general outpatient psychiatry, two thirds of patients on an antidepressant are on at least one other systemically taken, prescription medication. In fact, one third of all patients on an antidepressant are on three or more other systemically taken, prescription medications (Table 10.1).

These percentages are even higher in older and more medically ill populations. That fact has three consequences:

- Elderly and more medically ill patients are at greater risk for having a drug-drug interaction.

TABLE 10.1 — PERCENTAGE OF PATIENTS ON ANTIDEPRESSANTS HAVING THE POTENTIAL TO EXPERIENCE A DRUG-DRUG INTERACTION AS A FUNCTION OF TREATMENT SETTING

Clinical	Number of Patients	Prescribed Only an Antidepressant	Prescribed at Least One Other Medication	Prescribed Three or More Other Medications
Primary-care setting	2045	28%	72%	34%
Psychiatry clinic	224	29%	71%	30%
VA medical clinics	1076	7%	93%	68%
HIV clinic	66	2%	98%	77%

Abbreviations: VA, Veterans Administration; HIV, human immunodeficiency virus.

Other medications include a systemically taken, prescription drug from any therapeutic class. Does not include over-the-counter medications, topicals, or herbs.

Adapted from: Preskorn SH. *J Prac Psych Behav Hlth.* 1998;4:37-40.

- Due to their fragile health, any adverse outcome due to such an interaction is likely to be more serious.
- Finally, the interaction is more likely to be erroneously attributed to a worsening of their underlying health problems. Such a misattribution will likely delay effective intervention and can also increase health-care utilization (ie, increased use of laboratory tests to determine the cause of the problem). It can even increase the number of medications the patient is taking since the clinician may add another medication to treat what is, in fact, a drug-drug interaction.

The importance of this issue is further underscored by a literature search that revealed that the annual number of publications on drug-drug interactions increased five-fold from 1970 through 1997. Potential reasons include:
- Increases in both the number and type of medications available.
- An increase in the use of maintenance drug therapy for chronic conditions (eg, diabetes, hypertension, clinical depression).
- Increased percentage of elderly in the US population (these patients are likely to have one or more chronic illnesses which require concomitant drug therapy).

Patients with clinical depression may be particularly at risk for being on polydrug therapy for the following reasons:
- Patients with a variety of chronic medical illnesses have a higher incidence of clinical depression than physically healthy patients (Table 10.2). These patients will be on medications for their chronic medical conditions as well as on an antidepressant.

TABLE 10.2 — PREVALENCE OF MAJOR DEPRESSION IN SPECIFIC MEDICALLY ILL POPULATIONS

Medical Illness	Prevalence
Terminal solid tumors	25% to 38%
Stroke	27% to 35%
Renal disease	5% to 22%
Chronic pain	35% to > 50%
Epilepsy	20% to 30%
Parkinson's disease	30% to 50%
Myocardial infarction	20%
Diabetes mellitus	10%

Data from: Evans D. *Am Soc Clin Psychopharm Progress Notes.* 1995;6:22-25; Robertson MM, Trimble MR. *Epilepsia.* 1983;24(suppl 2):S109-S116; and Series HG. *J Psychosom Res.* 1992;36:1-16.

- Patients with clinical depression have a higher utilization of medical services in comparison to patients who are not depressed.
- Depressed patients often present with a variety of medical complaints (eg, headaches, muscle aches) which can lead to concomitant drug therapy.
- The clinician may use a second drug to either treat an adverse effect caused by an antidepressant or to boost its effectiveness (Chapter 11).

For all of these reasons, the prescriber must consider the potential for a drug-drug interaction when selecting an antidepressant for a depressed patient. There are two ways an antidepressant can interact with a coprescribed drug:

- Through its mechanism of action (ie, a pharmacodynamic interaction)
- Through its inhibition of a drug metabolizing CYP enzyme (ie, a pharmacokinetic interaction).[75,254]

Twenty years ago, clinicians were acutely aware of the risk of drug-drug interactions when prescribing antidepressants because their only options were tricyclic antidepressants (TCAs) and monoamine oxidase inhibitors (MAOIs). As outlined in Chapters 6 through 8, the pharmacology of these older antidepressants is such that they cause a number of different types of potentially serious pharmacodynamic drug-drug interactions when used in combination with other medications. For that reason, many practitioners twenty years ago were reluctant to use these antidepressants in elderly or medically ill patients.

In comparison to TCAs, most newer antidepressants have a much more limited number of pharmacologic actions. As explained in Chapter 6, that fact accounts for their better tolerability, wider therapeutic index, and a reduced risk of interacting pharmacodynamically with other coprescribed drugs. For these reasons, clinicians may have been lulled into a false sense of security. However, a number of the newer antidepressants can cause pharmacokinetic drug-drug interactions by virtue of their inhibition of drug-metabolizing cytochrome P450 (CYP) enzymes (Table 6.10).

Cytochrome P450 enzyme-mediated interactions are probably the most common type of pharmacokinetic drug-drug interaction. They are also the most easily misinterpreted type of drug-drug interaction because they can present in a myriad of ways, including:
- Dose-dependent toxicity
- Dose-dependent tolerability problems

- Decreased efficacy
- Withdrawal symptoms.

These interactions typically cause an increase or a decrease in the concentration-dependent effects of the drug whose metabolism was altered. Hence, the prescriber may attribute the adverse outcome to a problem of "sensitivity" or "resistance" on the part of the patient.[168,174]

Because our understanding of the mechanism underlying such interactions (ie, the inhibition of CYP enzymes) has increased dramatically over the last decade and because of their clinical importance, the remainder of this chapter will be devoted to some actual case examples that demonstrate the problems CYP enzyme-mediated drug-drug interactions can cause.

Case Studies

■ Case 1: Sudden Death in a 36-Year-Old Man

This patient presented to his clinician with a recurrent episode of major depression.[187] He was otherwise physically healthy based on medical history and physical examination. The patient stated he was in danger of losing his job because of poor performance resulting from his lack of energy and motivation.

His psychiatric history revealed that his depressive illness began in his early twenties. The current episode was his fourth and had begun approximately 3 months before he presented for care. According to the patient's medical history, he had responded to previous treatment with either a tertiary amine tricyclic antidepressant (TATCA) alone or a serotonin selective reuptake inhibitor (SSRI) alone, but the response had been incomplete and had taken considerable time.

Due to concerns about his job, the patient desperately wanted to feel better quickly. In response, his prescriber used an augmentation strategy; the combined use of a TCA and an SSRI (Chapter 11). He chose amitriptyline, 150 mg/day, and fluoxetine, 40 mg/day. The patient responded quickly with his only adverse effect being a mild dry mouth. However, several weeks later, the patient was found dead.

There was no evidence of foul play. An autopsy found no anatomical cause of death. The results of the analyses of postmortem blood samples revealed toxic levels of amitriptyline and its active metabolite, nortriptyline. The coroner signed this case out initially as a suicide.

Explanation

Suicide is an understandable conclusion in this case for several reasons. The high levels of amitriptyline and its metabolites indicate a drug overdose. This patient had several risk factors for suicide (Table 4.1). He had recurrent clinical depression which leads to death by suicide in 15% of cases and had been under considerable psychosocial stress.

However, there were also several factors against this interpretation including the absence of a suicide note, no missing pills from his amitriptyline prescription bottle, and no pill fragments in his stomach.

The definitive answer about the cause of death came by examining the relative ratio of amitriptyline to nortriptyline in the gastric contents, blood, and tissue samples taken at autopsy. Amitriptyline is converted into nortriptyline by CYP 2D6-mediated oxidative drug metabolism. After taking amitriptyline on a regular basis for a week or more, an equilibrium (steady-state) is reached between the central compartment (the blood) and deep compartments in the tissue. Once steady-state is reached, the ratio of amitriptyline to nortriptyline is the same in the deep tissue compartment as it is in the blood.

Since gastric fluid is produced from the plasma, it reflects the ratio of drug in the plasma unless it is distorted by what is consumed. In an acute overdose, the amitriptyline in his stomach would dissolve into the gastric fluid substantially distorting the amitriptyline to nortriptyline ratio. In fact, patients typically die from an acute cardiac arrest before all of the amitriptyline is absorbed. For these reasons, in an acute amitriptyline overdose we would expect that the highest ratio of amitriptyline to nortriptyline would be in the stomach fluid, next highest in the blood, and lowest in the deep compartments. In this case, the ratios in these three compartments were the same, proving that this patient did not die from an acute overdose.

When these facts were presented to the coroner years later, the death certificate was corrected to show death occurred as a result of a chronic, unintentional overdose of amitriptyline consistent with fluoxetine-induced inhibition of CYP 2D6. In fact, the functional dose of amitriptyline in this case was closer to 900 mg/day than to the prescribed dose of 150 mg/day due to the fluoxetine-induced decrease in amitriptyline clearance.[186]

A dose of 900 mg/day would be expected to produce toxic levels in almost all patients. The time course from starting the combined therapy to the patient's death is due to the fact that it takes several weeks for fluoxetine to accumulate and sufficiently inhibit the metabolism of amitriptyline. That is the reason why the prescriber must consider the long half-life of fluoxetine when starting or stopping fluoxetine.

■ Case 2: Severe Parkinsonism and Confusion in a 78-Year-Old Woman

This patient was in a nursing home for cognitive impairment and delusions.[136] The latter problem had been successfully treated with molindone, an intermediate potency antipsychotic medication, which she tolerated with only a mild, intermittent resting tremor. She then developed a depressive episode and was treated with the SSRI, paroxetine. Being aware of the issue of drug-drug interactions, her prescriber reduced the dose of molindone from 30 mg/day to 20 mg/day. Two weeks later, the patient had a prominent 3-cycle-per-second resting tremor, mask-like facies, cogwheel rigidity, and was unable to walk or care for herself.

The clinician attributed these problems to the worsening of underlying Parkinson's disease. As a result, he reduced the dose of molindone to 10 mg/day and added L-dopa/carbidopa and the anticholinergic drug, benztropine. Over the next several days, the patient developed a superimposed delirium. All of her medications were then discontinued and she gradually returned to her baseline status over the next 2 weeks.

Explanation

The metabolism of molindone has not been characterized; however, this case suggests that CYP 2D6 plays a major role. If that is correct, then the addition of paroxetine 20 mg/day would be expected to substantially increase her molindone levels. In other words, her clinician would have functionally increased her dose of molindone conceivably well beyond 30 mg/day even though he thought he had reduced the dose to 20 mg/day.

An increased accumulation of molindone would produce a greater degree of dopamine receptor blockade in her brain which in turn would have caused the development of marked parkinsonism. The failure to consider this possibility led to the misdiagnosis and the addition of the antiparkinsonian medications which caused her delirium. While benztropine is another drug whose metabolism has not been characterized, some authors have postulated a CYP 2D6 component on the basis of cases of delirium occurring following the addition of fluoxetine or paroxetine to patients on stable doses of benztropine.[11,211]

As in the first case, this example illustrates how "not seeing" may simply mean "not recognizing." It also shows how the adverse consequence of a drug-drug interaction can be mistaken for another disease. The result can be both poor patient outcome and increased health-care costs.

■ Case 3: A 44-Year-Old Man at Risk for Seizures

This patient had grand mal epilepsy and a triad of behavioral problems (irritability, angry outbursts, and agitation) for which he had been treated for some time with phenytoin, 400 mg/day, and carbamazepine, 600 mg/day.[224] On this regimen, he improved in terms of both seizure control and behavior. When he later presented with a major depressive episode, his prescriber added the SSRI, fluoxetine 20 mg/day. The depressive episode resolved. He also experienced a further reduction in the frequency of seizures and behavioral problems.

After 1 year of successful maintenance therapy, the fluoxetine was stopped since he had only one depressive episode. One month after discontinuation of the fluoxetine, his phenytoin level had fallen by 50% and was below the usually effective threshold for seizure control. His carbamazepine levels had also fallen, but only by approximately 15%.

Explanation

Fortunately, a quality-control program detected the potential problem. The alerted clinician rechecked the patient's phenytoin and carbamazepine levels and increased their dose. If that had not occurred, this patient was at risk for both an increase in his seizure frequency and a worsening of his behavioral problems.

In this case, the problem was a loss of the inhibitory effect of fluoxetine on the clearance of the anticonvulsants. During fluoxetine coadministration, the levels of the anticonvulsants had risen which likely accounted for the better control of his seizure disorder and behavioral problems during that time. However, the prescriber did not understand that he needed to increase the doses of the anticonvulsants when he stopped fluoxetine if he wanted to maintain these higher levels.

This case demonstrates that loss of efficacy can result from a CYP enzyme-mediated drug-drug interaction. It also illustrates that a drug like fluoxetine can have different effects on two CYP enzymes. CYP 2C9/10 mediates the metabolism of phenytoin and is substantially inhibited by fluoxetine 20 mg/day, while CYP 3A mediates the metabolism of carbamazepine and is only mildly inhibited by fluoxetine 20 mg/day (Tables 6.9 and 6.10).

Had this patient experienced a seizure, the clinician might have erroneously concluded that the patient had not been compliant when he found low anticonvulsant plasma levels on repeat therapeutic drug monitoring.

■ Case 4: The 28-Year-Old Man With Abdominal Cramps, Chills, and Runny Nose

This patient was a narcotic addict and had been successfully treated for several years with methadone.[24] He then developed a depressive episode that was in turn successfully treated with the SSRI, fluvoxamine, 200 mg/day. After 3 months, the clinician decided to stop the SSRI, feeling treatment was adequate. Within several days, this patient experienced abdominal cramps, loose stools, sweating, tremulousness, chills, and a runny nose.

Explanation

The patient was in narcotic withdrawal. The reason is that fluvoxamine produces substantial inhibition of CYP 1A2 which metabolizes methadone (Table 6.9). During the 3 months that this patient was on fluvoxamine, his methadone levels had risen as a result of decreased clearance and he had become dependent on the higher methadone levels. When the fluvoxamine was stopped, his methadone clearance increased and his methadone levels fell precipitating withdrawal symptoms.

Had the clinician not thought of this possibility, he might have thought the patient was drug seeking or that the symptoms were due to an intercurrent medical problem. The latter interpretation could have resulted in unnecessary medical testing while the patient suffered needlessly.

Summary

The information reviewed in these case studies should help demystify the issue of drug-drug interactions, particularly those mediated by CYP enzymes. The cases illustrate that CYP enzyme-mediated drug-drug interactions can present in myriad ways from sudden and life-threatening toxicity to more subtle but nevertheless clinically important problems. Such interactions can result in poor patient outcome and increased health-care costs, and frequently have the same consequence as would occur with a comparable change in the dose of the affected (or "victim") drug.

While this book is focused on antidepressant pharmacotherapy, the basic concepts covered in this chapter are relevant to all therapeutic classes of medications. By understanding the mechanisms underlying such interactions, clinicians can minimize the risk of such interactions by proper drug selection. Fortunately, there are a number of newer antidepressant options that generally do not produce clinically meaningful inhibition of drug metabolizing enzymes and hence are not at serious risk for causing such interactions (Table 6.10).

10

11
When the Patient Does Not Respond Well to Initial Antidepressant Therapy

Regrettably, no single antidepressant will produce an adequate response in every patient with clinical depression. Despite using all of the information summarized in the preceding chapter to make the best possible treatment selection, some patients will not respond because they do not tolerate the medication well enough to remain on it for an adequate period of time to respond. Others will simply have a form of the illness which is not responsive to the mechanism of action of the antidepressant. This chapter will present some simple and useful approaches to take when faced with such an outcome.

Some of the recommendations in this chapter will be to add a second medication either as an "antidote" for a treatment limiting adverse effect or as a means of boosting efficacy in a patient who has experienced an incomplete response. In essence, these approaches are planned drug-drug interactions and thus are the opposite side of the issue discussed in Chapter 10. Although such therapeutic drug-drug interactions can be quite clinically helpful when properly employed, they should only be used when monodrug therapy has failed to produce an acceptable response. The goal is always to keep treatment as simple and safe as possible.

The practitioner can use the pharmacological profiles of the various antidepressants discussed in Chapters 6 through 8 to optimally match the antidepressant to the patient. Nevertheless, adverse effects will occur despite the most careful selection. When the effect is serious and/or severe, the clinician can refer to Table 6.4 to determine what mechanism likely mediates the effect, and then use Table 6.3 to select an antidepressant which does not have that mechanism of action.

In many cases, the adverse effect will be a nuisance, but will not warrant a medication switch. Often, these adverse effects are dose dependent and a dose reduction may alleviate the problem. Moreover, tolerance occurs for many of the acute adverse effects of the antidepressants probably as a result of receptor down regulation. For this reason, the dose can be gradually re-escalated, if needed for optimal efficacy, without the adverse effect necessarily recurring. Treatment of the most common nuisance adverse effects of the various antidepressants (Tables 6.7 and 6.8) are discussed below.

■ Anorexia

This effect is most commonly mediated by indirect serotonin (5-hydroxytryptophan [5-HT]) agonism, probably of the 5-HT2C receptor, produced by the inhibition of serotonin uptake.[238] It occurs in a dose-dependent fashion with all serotonin selective reuptake inhibitors (SSRIs) and venlafaxine. Tolerance commonly develops.[103,171] Such tolerance is the reason these antidepressants were not able to show sustained weight loss when they were being tested as weight-reduction agents. If the anorexia persists and the clinician and patient do not want to switch to a

194

different type of antidepressant, then the addition of a 5-HT2C antagonists such as mirtazapine or cyproheptadine can be helpful.

■ Confusion

This effect can occur as a result of several mechanisms of action; principally, the blockade of the muscarinic acetylcholine, histamine-1, and 5-HT2A receptors.[83,193,220] It is dose dependent. Tolerance frequently does not develop. There is no good antidote.

■ Constipation

This effect is most commonly seen with antidepressants that block the muscarinic acetylcholine receptor, but may also occur with norepinephrine uptake inhibitors. It is dose dependent. Tolerance frequently does not develop when it is caused by muscarinic acetylcholine receptor blockade. Bulk forming stool softeners can be used to minimize the problem.

■ Diaphoresis

This effect is most commonly seen with antidepressants that inhibit norepinephrine uptake. It is frequently not dose dependent. Tolerance often does not occur. Beta blockers can be helpful in some cases.

■ Diarrhea

Loose or frequent stools is a better descriptor. This effect occurs in a dose-dependent fashion with all SSRIs and venlafaxine. Tolerance commonly develops. Drugs which slow gut motility can be helpful, such as lomotil or anticholinergics.

■ Dizziness

This term is often used to describe two different effects: one associated with decreased peripheral vascular resistance as a result of alpha-1–adrenergic receptor blockade and one due to direct or indirect 5-HT1A stimulation.[83] The former is clinically more important than the latter because it is more likely to be associated with loss of balance leading to falls, and is more likely to be persistent. There is no good antidote besides dose reduction. When only tricyclic antidepressants (TCAs) were available, clinicians would recommend increasing the salt intake and the use of thromboembolic disease hose; these steps can be helpful in some cases. Falls can be minimized by instructing patients to slowly change from lying to sitting and then to standing to allow accommodation to occur.

The dizziness caused by 5-HT1A stimulation is most likely centrally mediated. It can occur early in treatment with antidepressants which inhibit serotonin uptake (eg, SSRIs and venlafaxine) and/or block 5-HT2A receptors (eg, nefazodone and mirtazapine) as well as drugs which directly stimulate the 5-HT1A receptor (eg, buspirone). There are no cardiovascular changes associated with it. Balance and coordination are subjectively, but not objectively, affected. Tolerance commonly develops within days to a week. While it is not medically serious, it can be disturbing if the patient has not been forewarned about this potential adverse effect.

■ Drowsiness

This effect can occur as a result of several mechanisms of action, principally the blockade of the histamine-1 and 5-HT2A receptors and serotonin reuptake inhibition.[83,220] It is generally more severe, persistent, and dose dependent when caused by histamine-1 receptor blockade. When the pharmacokinetics of the drugs permit (ie, half-life of approximately 1 day), the majority, if not all, of the dose can be given at night which can help with sleep and reduce, if not eliminate, daytime sedation.

196

As discussed in Chapter 8, there are some reasons to believe that this effect of mirtazapine may follow a curvilinear dose-response curve (ie, the effect diminishes with higher doses). The presumed mechanism is the offsetting arousal effect that can occur with the alpha-2–adrenergic receptor blockade produced by higher doses of mirtazapine (Figure 6.4).

■ Dry Mouth

This effect is most commonly seen with antidepressants that block the muscarinic acetylcholine receptor, but may also occur with norepinephrine uptake inhibitors. It is dose dependent. Tolerance frequently does not develop when caused by muscarinic acetylcholine receptor blockade. While it is frequently considered a trivial or nuisance adverse effect, it can result in increased tooth decay and gum disease due to the loss of the bacteriostatic effects of saliva. Patients should be advised to practice excellent dental hygiene, including brushing after every meal, avoiding snacks (particularly those which are sweet), and flossing. Chewing sugarless gum can be helpful.

■ Fatigue

This term is frequently used interchangeably with drowsiness and tiredness in clinical trial reporting. However, these terms are not necessarily synonymous. Fatigue can be a persistent symptom of an incompletely treated depressive episode. In other instances, it can be due to the type of disturbed sleep characteristically produced by serotonin reuptake inhibitors (SRIs) (ie, decreased rapid eye movement [REM], sleep and a shift from stage IV deep, restorative sleep to light stage I sleep).[9,159,217,226,230] Paradoxically, patients with decreased REM sleep may report an increase in vivid dreaming since they are more likely to awaken during or near an REM interval as a result of the shift to light stage I sleep. For this type of day-time fatigue, the use of a 5-HT2A blocker such as trazodone can be helpful or the use of a short-lived benzodiazepine such as lorazepam to restore more normal sleep efficiency and restorative value.[155]

■ Hyperphagia

Although this effect was thought to be due to his-tamine-1 receptor blockade, it is more likely the re-sult of 5-HT2C blockade which can be produced by antidepressants such as mirtazapine.[83] Dose reduction is usually not helpful. Tolerance develops less fre-quently than with other adverse effects of antidepres-sants (eg, nausea). There are no truly effective anti-dotes. Instead, switching to another antidepressant is frequently necessary.

■ Insomnia

Initial insomnia can be either a persistent depres-sive symptom or an adverse effect of a more stimu-lating antidepressant such as a norepinephrine and/or dopamine reuptake inhibitor (eg, desipramine or bupropion, respectively). In the latter case, the ap-proach is to move more of the dose to earlier in the day. Nevertheless, bupropion still must be given on a divided schedule as discussed in Chapter 8. Middle or late insomnia is more likely due to the disruptive effects that serotonin agonism can have on sleep ar-chitecture and is treated as discussed above under the section on fatigue.[159,217,226,230]

■ Nausea

This effect is most commonly mediated by indi-rect 5-HT3 agonism resulting from the inhibition of serotonin uptake.[83] It occurs in a dose-dependent fash-ion with all SSRIs and venlafaxine. Tolerance typi-cally develops. Cisapride can be used to block this effect when necessary,[23] but it should not be used with antidepressants that produce substantial inhibition of the drug metabolizing cytochrome P450 (CYP) enzyme 3A (ie, fluvoxamine, nefazodone and high doses of fluoxetine) (Table 6.10).

■ Nervousness

This effect can occur as a result of the inhibition of the uptake pumps for norepinephrine and to a lesser extent serotonin. It is dose dependent. Tolerance may not develop. Beta blockers can be helpful in some patients. Benzodiazepines may also be used, but carry a modest risk for abuse and/or dependence.

■ Sexual Dysfunction

This effect is most commonly mediated by indirect serotonin agonism produced by the inhibition of serotonin uptake. It occurs in a dose-dependent fashion with all SSRIs and venlafaxine.[145,147] Unlike most of the other adverse effects discussed here, this one typically occurs only after several weeks of treatment. Tolerance frequently does not develop.

Although many possible antidotes have been tried, no single effective approach has emerged. All of the following have been tried with varying degrees of success: buspirone (Buspar), bupropion (Wellbutrin), cyproheptadine (Periactin), yohimbine (Aphrodyne, Erex, Yocon, Yohimex), sildenafil (Viagra), and topically applied 1% testosterone creams for anorgasmia in women. The best antidote may be dopamine agonism produced by the addition of bupropion or methylphenidate. However, caution must be used with the dose of bupropion, particularly when used in conjunction with antidepressants that produce substantial inhibition of the drug metabolizing CYP enzymes (Table 6.10) as discussed in Chapter 6.

■ **Vision Disturbance**

This term is used to describe two different effects. The first is visual trails most likely caused by 5-HT receptor blockade.[83] The second is impaired accommodation caused by the blockade of the muscarinic acetylcholine receptor. Visual trails are also referred to as "after images." Nefazodone is the antidepressant which is most likely to cause visual trails (Table 6.8). While it is not serious, some patients may be alarmed by its occurrence if not prewarned. Tolerance may develop in the case of both visual trails and accommodation. There are no established antidotes for either adverse effect.

Special notes: Dose-dependent adverse effects produced by serotonin reuptake inhibition can occur later in treatment and persist longer with fluoxetine than with the other SSRIs due to the long half-lives of the parent drug and its active metabolite, norfluoxetine.[168] The clinician should keep this issue in mind when managing patients on this SSRI.

There are other, less frequent adverse effects and also more complicated management approaches than those discussed here. However, they are beyond what many primary-care practitioners would use in their practice. In such cases, referral to a psychiatrist who specializes in more complicated drug management may be the best course of action.

Partial Response

Partial response means that there has been at least a 25% improvement in the patient's symptomatology. While the patient is better, they are still symptomatic to a clinically significant extent. The clinician can quantitate the severity of the episode either by clinical interview or by the use of a patient self-reporting scale such as the Zung Depression Self-Report Rating Scale (Figure 9.2). The improvement in the depressive syndrome may be in one or more of the following areas:

- Mood
- Sleep
- Appetite
- Energy
- Sex drive
- Interest
- Concentration/attention.

The areas that have improved are often dependent on the class of antidepressant used. For example, SRIs may produce more improvement in irritability, interest, and concentration/attention, while TCAs, nefazodone, and mirtazapine will often produce more improvement in sleep and appetite.[103]

■ Dose Adjustment

If the depressive episode has had a partial response but not a full remission after a 4-week trial, then a dose increase with all of the antidepressants except TCAs is a reasonable approach. This recommendation even holds true for the SSRIs despite their flat dose-response curve because the patient may be a rapid metabolizer and hence may develop plasma drug levels too low for an optimal response.[170] The patient should receive a 4-week trial of this higher dose, assuming that his/her condition is improved sufficiently to warrant this disciplined approach and that s/he is agreeable to it. In the case of TCAs, the dose should have already been optimized based on therapeutic drug monitoring as discussed in Chapter 8. If the patient has had a partial response after 4 weeks of treatment with a TCA at therapeutic plasma drug levels, then a dose change is not warranted.[191] Instead, the patient should be maintained on this dose for an additional 2 weeks to assess whether there will be any further response to this drug.

■ Augmentation Strategies

Another approach is augmentation strategies.[244] The concept behind such strategies is a planned drug-drug interaction (Chapter 10). Unfortunately, the amount of systematic and controlled data supporting the usefulness and long-term safety of these approaches are modest. The data that exist are not as robust as initially suggested by case reports and anecdotal clinical literature. Nevertheless, such strategies may be beneficial and are frequently tried in psychiatric practices when dealing with patients in whom other approaches have not worked.

The potential advantages of such strategies include:

- Conversion of partial responders to responders without having to start a new medication trial, and thus hopefully saving time and thus reducing patient suffering
- At times, lower doses of one or both agents may be sufficient, minimizing the likelihood of adverse effects
- The second drug may also treat a comorbid condition (eg, subclinical thyroid dysfunction).

The potential disadvantages stem from the fact that two agents are being used rather than one, and this increases the possibility of:

- Adverse effects
- Noncompliance
- Expense.

The most frequent augmentation strategies involve the addition of lithium, thyroid hormone, or psychostimulants to antidepressants. More recently, agents such as pindolol and buspirone have also been tried.

Lithium

The addition of lithium is perhaps the best studied and most popular augmentation strategy.[97,152,212] Improvement is often reported within a few days to weeks of adding lithium. The dose of lithium used in this strategy (ie, 450 to 600 mg/day) is generally lower than that used for the treatment of acute mania or prophylaxis of bipolar disorder.[231] Similarly, plasma lithium levels are lower in the range of 0.4 to 0.8 mEq/L. Added expense is minimal.

Thyroid Supplementation

There is a large body of literature outlining a strong association between clinical thyroid disease and psychiatric syndromes, especially mood disorders.[68] Over the past 25 years, evidence has accumulated suggesting T3 augmentation of partial or nonresponders with major depression can be a useful clinical strategy.[106] T3 (dosage range of 25 to 75 mg/day) is generally the preferred agent in the literature rather than a comparable dose of T4. The literature suggests that 50% to 60% of patients will benefit. One carefully controlled study comparing thyroid versus lithium augmentation found them to be equally efficacious.[106]

Crucial questions of biochemical and/or clinical predictors, dose-effect relationship, what constitutes an adequate trial, duration of treatment and long-term adverse effects have not been answered. However, the ease of use, the modest risk of untoward adverse drug-hormone interactions, and the administration of doses that are unlikely to effect the hypothalamic pituitary axis are factors that make this a useful strategy. Added expense is also minimal.

Psychostimulants/Dopamine Agonists (methylphenidate and d-amphetamine)

Like bupropion, these drugs may be useful as monodrug therapy for certain patients with apathy and/

or clinical depression associated with cerebrovascular accidents, Parkinson's disease and cancer. Their advantages include:

- Relative safety
- Rapidity of onset.

Their adverse effects can include:

- Anxiety
- Agitation
- Rarely psychosis
- Possible worsening of hypertension
- Abuse/addictive potential in some patients.

These drugs may also be useful as augmenting agents in the treatment of depressive disorders.[30,103] Dopamine agonists such as bromocriptine and pergolide have also been used as augmenting agents, but there is even less data supporting the efficacy and safety of such a combination. Added expense is more of an issue than with lithium and thyroid supplementation, but is still relatively modest.

Pindolol

Pindolol is a beta blocker and a 5-HT1A receptor antagonist which has recently been studied as a potentiating agent.[27,149] Some open-label and controlled studies have reported a more rapid response and perhaps greater efficacy when pindolol is added to an SRI to treat patients with major depression. The presumed mechanism involves interruption in the short-loop negative feedback system, allowing for an increase in synaptic concentrations of 5-HT. Added expense is modest.

Buspirone

Buspirone is a partial 5-HT1A agonist marketed in the 1980s as an anxiolytic agent. There is some evidence suggesting that it may have weak intrinsic antidepressant properties. It has recently been promoted as possibly being useful as an augmenting strategy, particularly with SRIs.[235] Neither the time of onset of action nor the optimal dose for augmentation has been rigorously established. When used as monodrug therapy for anxiety disorder, the dose is usually 15 to 30 mg/day and the time to onset is several weeks. Advantages of this augmentation strategy include its safety, the possible anxiolytic effects in the absence of abuse potential, and ease of use. Its principal disadvantage beyond limited data is cost. It is the most expensive of the augmentation strategies discussed in this section. Given that buspirone is still a patented drug, there will hopefully be more rigorous clinical trials to determine the relative merits of using this agent as an antidepressant augmentor.

Failed Trial

By definition, this term means that there has been less than a 25% change in depressive symptoms. In such cases, approaches other than those discussed above are generally recommended. The issue of what to do in such cases is arguably the greatest research need in antidepressant pharmacotherapy, but is disappointingly sparse.[98,157,215,246] The existing studies have serious limitations such as small numbers of subjects and design problems, including no blinding, no random assignment, and no appropriate control group.

■ Alternative Monodrug Therapy
Some clinicians will try multiple members of the same class (eg, multiple sequential trials of different SSRIs) in patients who have not experienced adequate benefit. An argument can be made from a pharmacokinetic standpoint that a trial of a second SSRI might

be a reasonable approach. Unfortunately, the studies that have been done to support this practice are all seriously flawed and thus of dubious merit.[37,105,182,242] Certainly, the more rational approach after two SSRIs have failed would be switching to an antidepressant with a different presumed mechanism of action (Table 6.2).

The best data in this area come from double-blind, crossover studies which show that norepinephrine selective reuptake inhibitors (NSRIs) will work in approximately 50% of patients who have not benefited from an adequate trial of an SSRI and vice versa.[103,245] Another approach is to escalate the dose of a drug with more than one antidepressant mechanism of action (eg, venlafaxine).[156,177] For further discussion of this matter, refer to Chapters 6 through 8.

■ Copharmacy With Antidepressants

When two or more trials of monodrug therapy with antidepressants from different classes have failed to produce even a partial response, the most common approach is to use two chemically unrelated antidepressants in combination.[245] This strategy is based more on clinical empiricism and a theoretical understanding of relevant neurotransmitter systems than on rigorous clinical trials. The earliest example of this strategy was the combined use of a TCA and an MAOI.[103] With the introduction of safer antidepressants, the use of this specific combination has decreased due to concerns about toxicity. However, the use of other combinations of antidepressants has increased in terms of both frequency and the variety of combinations used. The most popular is the combined use of an SSRI (eg, sertraline) with an NSRI (eg, desipramine) or with a dopamine and norepinephrine reuptake inhibitor (eg, bupropion).[153,258]

The following points should be kept in mind when considering this option:

206

- They are planned drug-drug interactions (Chapter 10) with the potential for increased adverse effects, the likely need to reduce the dose, and the need for even more careful monitoring, including therapeutic drug monitoring (TDM).
- These strategies should be attempted in a systematic and well documented manner; patients should be well informed.
- Certain combinations must be avoided such as an SSRI plus MAOI due to the potentially fatal serotonin syndrome.

Specific Combination Treatments for Special Patients

Some patients with specific types of clinical depression may need specific combination treatment strategies, such as:
- Antidepressant plus anxiolytic
- Antidepressant plus antipsychotic
- Antidepressant plus mood stabilizer.

■ Antidepressant Plus Anxiolytic

There are patients with prominent anxiety and depressive symptoms (ie, mixed anxiety and depression).[190] Ideally, monodrug therapy, preferably an antidepressant with proven efficacy in anxiety disorders, should be tried first (Table 8.2). When using this approach, it is advisable to start with a low dose of the antidepressant because a variety of antidepressants can cause nervousness (Chapter 6), and anxious patients may be particularly vulnerable to this adverse effect. If the patient experiences an increase in anxiety despite starting with a low dose, the combined use of the antidepressant plus anxiolytic (eg, clonazepam) can be used. After the antidepressant has had time to exert its full antidepressant effects (2 to 4 weeks), an attempt can be made to taper and stop the anxiolytic medication. There is a small percentage of patients in whom anxiety symptoms will recur when the anxiolytic is stopped, even though they have a full resolution of their depressive symptoms. Such patients may need indefinite combined treatment with an antidepressant and anxiolytic, but the goal would be to have such combined treatment be the exception rather than the rule.[235]

■ Antidepressants Plus Antipsychotics

There are also patients who have both depressive and psychotic symptoms (eg, mood congruent hallucinations or delusions). Such a presentation may lead to a false positive diagnosis of schizophrenia which, in turn, can result in treatment with antipsychotics alone. That may alleviate the psychotic symptoms but not address the underlying mood disorder. Conversely, there are patients with subtle forms of delusions such as a nihilistic delusion ("I have never been any good" or "I am financially ruined") which may be missed. When treated with an antidepressant alone, these patients often do not improve. A better strategy for such patients is combined treatment with an antidepressant and an antipsychotic or alternatively electroconvulsive therapy.[103]

■ Antidepressants Plus Mood Stabilizers

As discussed in Chapter 1, patients with bipolar (ie, manic-depressive) disorder may present for the first time clinically in the depressed phase of their illness. If there is a past personal (or family) history of unequivocal hypomania or mania, treating with an antidepressant alone may increase the likelihood of a manic episode. In such patients, the use of a mood stabilizer (eg, lithium, valproate) alone or in combination with an antidepressant is a preferable course of action. In fact, there is some evidence that lithium can be effective as monodrug therapy for mild depressive episodes.

■ Electroconvulsive Therapy

Electroconvulsive therapy (ECT) remains the single most effective treatment for clinical depression and remains an important treatment option for the severely depressed patient or the patient who has not benefited from antidepressant therapy.[103,216] A recently developed and still investigational treatment is repetitive transcranial magnetic stimulation (rTMS) which involves the depolarization of neurons in a localized area of the brain by applying a powerful magnetic field in rapid flux.[22]

11

12 References

1. Adler LA, Angrist BM. Paroxetine and akathisia. *Biol Psychiatry*. 1995;37:336-337.

2. Alderman CP, Seshadri P, Ben-Tovim DI. Effects of serotonin reuptake inhibitors on hemostasis. *Ann Pharmacother*. 1996;30:1232-1234.

3. American Academy of Child and Adolescent Psychiatry. Practice parameters for the assessment and treatment of children and adolescents with obsessive-compulsive disorder. *J Am Acad Child Adolesc Psychiatry*. 1998;37(suppl 10):275-455.

4. American Psychiatric Association. Practice guidelines for major depressive disorder in adults. *Am J Psychiatry*. 1993;150(suppl 4):1-26.

5. Amsterdam JD, Garcia-Espana F, Goodman D, Hooper M, Hornig-Rohan M. Breast enlargement during chronic antidepressant therapy. *J Affect Disord*. 1997;46:151-156.

6. Andreasen NC, Rice J, Endicott J, Coryell W, Grove WM, Reich T. Familial rates of affective disorder. A report from the National Institute of Mental Health Collaborative Study [published erratum appears in *Arch Gen Psychiatry*. 1988;45:776]. *Arch Gen Psychiatry*. 1987;44:461-469.

7. Anonymous. Drugs for psychiatric disorders. *Med Lett Drugs Ther*. 1994;36:89-96.

8. Arana GW, Baldessarini RJ, Ornsteen M. The dexamethasone suppression test for diagnosis and prognosis in psychiatry. Commentary and review. *Arch Gen Psychiatry*. 1985;42:1193-1204.

9. Armitage R, Trivedi M, Rush AJ. Fluoxetine and oculomotor activity during sleep in depressed patients. *Neuropsychopharmacology*. 1995;12:159-165.

10. Armitage R, Rush AJ, Trivedi M, Cain J, Roffwarg HP. The effects of nefazodone on sleep architecture in depression. *Neuropsychopharmacology*. 1994;10:123-127.

11. Armstrong SC, Schweitzer SM. Delirium associated with paroxetine and benztropine combination. *Am J Psychiatry*. 1997;154:581-582. Letter.

12. Aronson TA, Shukla S, Hoff A, Cook B. Proposed delusional depression subtypes: preliminary evidence from a retrospective study of phenomenology and treatment course. *J Affect Disord*. 1988;14:69-74.

13. Ayd FJ. Paroxetine, a new selective serotonin reuptake inhibitor. *Int Drug Ther Newsletter*. 1993;28:5-12.

14. Baldassano CF, Truman CJ, Nierenberg A, Ghaemi SN, Sachs GS. Akathisia: a review and case report following paroxetine treatment. *Compr Psychiatry*. 1996;37:122-124.

15. Baldwin D, Fineberg N, Montgomery S. Fluoxetine, fluvoxamine and extrapyramidal tract disorders. *Int Clin Psychopharmacol*. 1991;6:51-58.

16. Balon R. Antidepressants in the treatment of premature ejaculation. *J Sex Marital Ther*. 1996;22:85-96.

17. Barker EL, Blakely RD. Norepinephrine and serotonin transporters: molecular targets of antidepressant drugs. In: Bloom FE, Kupfer DJ, eds. *Psychopharmacology: The Fourth Generation of Progress*. New York, NY: Raven Press; 1994;321-334.

18. Barr LC, Goodman WK, Price LH. Physical symptoms associated with paroxetine discontinuation. *Am J Psychiatry*. 1994;151:289. Letter.

19. Bayer AJ, Roberts NA, Allen EA, et al. The pharmacokinetics of paroxetine in the elderly. *Acta Psychiatr Scand*. 1989;350(suppl):85-86.

20. Beasley CM, Masica DN, Heiligenstein JH, et al. Possible monoamine oxidate inhibitor—serotonin uptake inhibitor interaction: fluoxetine clinical data and preclinical findings. *J Clin Psychopharmacol*. 1993;13:312-320.

21. Beck AT, Brown G, Berchick RJ, Stewart BL, Steer RA. Relationship between hopelessness and ultimate suicide: a replication with psychiatric outpatients. *Am J Psychiatry*. 1990;147:190-195.

22. Beedle D, Krasuski J, Janicak PG. Advances in somatic therapies: electroconvulsive therapy, repetitive transcranial magnetic stimulation and bright light therapy. In: Janicak PG, Davis JM, Preskorn SH, Ayd FJ, eds. *Principles and Practice of Psychopharmacotherapy*. 2nd ed. Baltimore, Md: Lippincott, Williams & Wilkins; 1998:1-170.

23. Bergeron R, Blier P. Cisapride for the treatment of nausea produced by selective serotonin reuptake inhibitors. *Am J Psychiatry*. 1994;151:1084-1086.

24. Bertschy G, Baumann P, Eap CB, Baettig D. Probable metabolic interaction between methadone and fluvoxamine in addict patients. *Ther Drug Monit*. 1994;16:42-45.

25. Bhatara VS, Bandettini FC. Possible interaction between sertraline and tranylcypromine. *Clin Pharmacol*. 1993;12: 222-225.

26. Blayac JP, Hillaire-Buys D, Peyrière H. Pharmacovigilance of new antidepressants: evaluation of neuro-psychobehavioral disorders [in French]. *Therapie*. 1997;52:117-122.

27. Blier P, Bergeron R. The use of pindolol to potentiate antidepressant medication. *J Clin Psychiatry*. 1998;59(suppl 5):16-23, 24-25.

28. Bloch M, Stager SV, Braun AR, Rubinow DR. Severe psychiatric symptoms associated with paroxetine withdrawal. *Lancet*. 1995;346:57. Letter.

29. Blume CD. Dear doctor letter regarding use of eldepryl. Tampa, Fla: Somerset Pharmaceuticals; 1994, Nov 14.

30. Bodkin JA, Lasser RA, Wines JD Jr, Gardner DM, Baldessarini RJ. Combining serotonin reuptake inhibitors and bupropion in partial responders to antidepressant monotherapy. *J Clin Psychiatry*. 1997;58:137-145.

31. Bolden-Watson C, Richelson E. Blockade by newly-developed antidepressants of biogenic amine uptake into rat brain synaptosomes. *Life Sci*. 1993;52:1023-1029.

32. Brannan SK, Talley BJ, Bowden CL. Sertraline and isocarboxazid cause a serotonin syndrome. *J Clin Psychopharmacol*. 1994;14:144-145. Letter.

33. Bremner JD, Wingard P, Walshe TA. Safety of mirtazapine in overdose. *J Clin Psychiatry*. 1998;59:233-235.

34. Broadhead WE, Blazer DG, George LK, Tse CK. Depression, disability days, and days lost from work in a prospective epidemiologic survey. *JAMA*. 1990;264:2524-2528.

35. Brown GW, Harris TO. *Social Origins of Depression:A Study of Psychiatric Disorder in Women*. London, UK: Tamstock Publications; 1978.

36. Brown WA, Dornseif BE, Wernicke JF. Placebo response in depression: a search for predictors. *Psychiatry Res*. 1988;26: 259-264.

37. Brown WA, Harrison W. Are patients who are intolerant to one SSRI intolerant to another? *Psychopharmcol Bull.* 1992;28:253-256.

38. Bryois C, Rubin C, Zbinden JD, Baumann P. Withdrawal syndrome caused by selective serotonin reuptake inhibitors: apropos of a case [in French]. *Schweiz Rundsch Med Prax.* 1998;87:345-348.

39. Bunney WE Jr, Goodwin FK, Murphy DL, House KM, Gordon EK. The "switch process" in manic-depressive illness. II. Relationship to catecholamines, REM sleep, and drugs. *Arch Gen Psychiatry.* 1972;27:304-309.

40. Burke MJ, Silkey B, Preskorn SH. Pharmacoeconomic considerations when evaluating treatment options for major depressive disorder. *J Clin Psychiatry.* 1994;55(suppl A):42-52, 53-54, 98-100.

41. Burrows GD, Maguire KP, Norman TR. Antidepressant efficacy and tolerability of the selective norepinephrine reuptake inhibitor reboxetine: a review. *J Clin Psychiatry.* 1998;59 (suppl 14):4-7.

42. Caccia S, Ballabio M, Samanin R, Zanini MG, Garattini S. (--)-m-Chlorophenylpiperazine, a central 5-hydroxytryptamine agonist, is a metabolite of trazodone. *J Pharm Pharmacol.* 1981;33:477-478.

43. Carpenter LL, McDougle CJ, Epperson CN, Price LH. A risk-benefit assessment of drugs used in the management of obsessive-compulsive disorder. *Drug Saf.* 1996;15:116-134.

44. Celexa (citalopram hydrobromide) [package insert]. St. Louis, Mo: Forest Pharmaceuticals, Inc; 1998.

45. Choo V. Paroxetine and extrapyramidal reactions. *Lancet.* 1993;341:624. Letter.

46. Chouinard G. Sertraline in the treatment of obsessive compulsive disorder: two double-blind, placebo-controlled studies. *Int Clin Psychopharmacol.* 1992;7(suppl 2):37-41.

47. Claghorn JL, Feighner JP. A double-blind comparison of paroxetine with imipramine in the long-term treatment of depression. *J Clin Psychopharmacol.* 1993;13(suppl 2):23S-27S.

48. Clerc GE, Ruimy P, Verdeau-Pallès J. A double-blind comparison of venlafaxine and fluoxetine in patients hospitalized for major depression and melancholia. The Venlafaxine French Inpatient Study Group. *Int Clin Psychopharmacol.* 1994;9:139-143.

49. Committee on Safety of Drugs. *Curr Prob Pharmaco-vigilance*. 1993;19:1.

50. Cooper TA, Valcour VG, Gibbons RB, O'Brien-Falls K. Spontaneous ecchymoses due to paroxetine administration. *Am J Med*. 1998;104:197-198.

51. Coplan JD, Gorman JM. Detectable levels of fluoxetine metabolites after discontinuation: an unexpected serotonin syndrome. *Am J Psychiatry*. 1993;150:837.

52. Costa e Silva J. Randomized, double-blind comparison of venlafaxine and fluoxetine in outpatients with major depression. *J Clin Psychiatry*. 1998;59:352-357.

53. Coupland NJ, Bell CJ, Potokar JP. Serotonin reuptake inhibitor withdrawal. *J Clin Psychopharmacol*. 1996;16:356-362.

54. Cusack B, Nelson A, Richelson E. Binding of antidepressants to human brain receptors: focus on newer generation compounds. *Psychopharmacology*. 1994;114:559-565.

55. Danish University Antidepressant Group. Citalopram: clinical effect profile in comparison with clomipramine. A controlled multicenter study. *Psychopharmacology*. 1986;90:131-138.

56. Danish University Antidepressant Group. Paroxetine: a selective serotonin reuptake inhibitor showing better tolerance, but weaker antidepressant effect than clomipramine in a controlled multicenter study. *J Affect Disord*. 1990;18:289-299.

57. Davidson J. Seizures and bupropion: a review. *J Clin Psychiatry*. 1989;50:256-261.

58. de Boer T, Ruigt G, Berendsen H. The alpha2-selective adrenoceptor antagonist Org 3770 (mirtazapine remeron) enhances noradrenergic and serotonergic transmission. *Hum Psychopharmacol*. 1995;10:107S-118S.

59. de Boer TH, Maura G, Raiteri M, de Vos CJ, Wieringa J, Pinder RM. Neurochemical and autonomic pharmacological profiles of the 6-aza-analogue of mianserin, Org 3770 and its enantiomers. *Neuropharmacology*. 1988;27:399-408.

60. Dechant KL, Clissold SP. Paroxetine. A review of its pharmacodynamic and pharmacokinetic properties, and therapeutic potential in depressive illness. *Drugs*. 1991;41:225-253.

61. Depression Guideline Panel. *Clinical Practice Guideline. Number 5. Depression in Primary Care, Vol. 1: Detection and Diagnosis*; and *Vol 2: Treatment of Major Depression.* Rockville, Md: US Dept. of Health and Human Services, Public Health Service, AHCPR Publication No. 93-0551; April, 1993.

62. Doogan DP, Caillard V. Sertraline in the prevention of depression. *Br J Psychiatry.* 1992;160:217-222.

63. *DSM-IV: Diagnostic and Statistical Manual of Mental Disorders.* 4th ed. Washington, DC: American Psychiatric Press; 1994.

64. Dunner DL, Gershon ES, Goodwin FK. Heritable factors in the severity of affective illness. *Biol Psychiatry.* 1976;11:31-42.

65. Effexor XR (venlafaxine hydrochloride) Extended-Release Capsules. In: *Physicians' Desk Reference.* 53rd ed. Montvale, NJ: Medical Economics Company, Inc; 1999:3298-3302.

66. Eldepryl (selegiline hydrochloride). In: *Physicians' Desk Reference.* 53rd ed. Montvale, NJ: Medical Economics Company, Inc; 1999:3128-3131.

67. Eric L. A prospective double-blind comparative multicentre study of paroxetine and placebo in preventing recurrent major depressive episodes. *Biol Psychiatry.* 1991;29(suppl 11):2545.

68. Esposito S, Prange AJ Jr, Golden RN. The thyroid axis and mood disorders: overview and future prospects. *Psychopharmacol Bull.* 1997;33:205-217.

69. Evans D. Antidepressant adverse effects and antidepressants in the medically ill. *Am Soc Clin Psychopharm Progress Notes.* 1995;6:22-25.

70. Evans ME, Kortas KJ. Potential interaction between isoniazid and selective serotonin-reuptake inhibitors. *Am J Health Syst Pharm.* 1995;52:2135-2136. Letter.

71. Fawcett J, Marcus RN, Anton SF, O'Brien K, Schwiderski U. Response of anxiety and agitation symptoms during nefazodone treatment of major depression. *J Clin Psychiatry.* 1995;56(suppl 6):37-42.

72. Fawcett J, Scheftner W, Clark D, Hedeker D, Gibbons R, Coryell W. Clinical predictors of suicide in patients with major affective disorders: a controlled prospective study. *Am J Psychiatry.* 1987;144:35-40.

73. Feighner JP. Cardiovascular safety in depressed patients: focus on venlafaxine. *J Clin Psychiatry*. 1995;56:574-579.

74. Feighner JP, Boyer WF, Tyler DL, Neborsky RJ. Adverse consequences of fluoxetine-MAOI combination therapy. *J Clin Psychiatry*. 1990;51:222-225.

75. Flockhart DA. Drug interactions, cardiac toxicity, and terfenadine: from bench to clinic? *J Clin Psychopharmacol*. 1996;16:101-103.

76. Frank E, Kupfer DJ, Perel JM, et al. Three-year outcomes for maintenance therapies in recurrent depression. *Arch Gen Psychiatry*. 1990;47:1093-1099.

77. Frazer A. Antidepressants. *J Clin Psychiatry*. 1997;58(suppl 6):9-25.

78. Frost L, Lal S. Shock-like sensations after discontinuance of selective serotonin reuptake inhibitors. *Am J Psychiatry*. 1995;152:810. Letter.

79. Garnier R, Azoyan P, Chataigner D, Taboulet P, Dellattre D, Efthymiou ML. Acute fluvoxamine poisoning. *J Int Med Res*. 1993;21:197-208.

80. Gershon ES, Berrettini W, Numberger J Jr, Goldin LR. Genetics of affective illness. In: Meltzer HY, ed. *Psychopharmacology: The Third Generation of Progress*. New York, NY: Raven Press; 1987:481-491.

81. Giammusso B, Morgia G, Spampinato A, Motta M. Paroxetine in the treatment of premature ejaculation [in Italian]. *Arch Ital Urol Androl*. 1997;69:11-13.

82. Gillin JC, Rapaport M, Erman MK, Winokur A, Albala BJ. A comparison of nefazodone and fluoxetine on mood and on objective, subjective, clinician-rated measures of sleep in depressed patients: a double-blind, 8-week clinical trial [published erratum appears in *J Clin Psychiatry*. 1997;58:275]. *J Clin Psychiatry*. 1997;58:185-192.

83. Glennon RA, Dukat M. Serotonin receptor subtypes. In: Bloom FE, Kupfer DJ, eds. *Psychopharmacology: The Fourth Generation of Progress*. New York, NY: Raven Press; 1994: 415-430.

84. Gonzalez FJ, Skoda RC, Kimura S, et al. Characterization of the common genetic defect in humans deficient in debrisoquine metabolism. *Nature*. 1988;331:442-446.

85. Goodwin DW, Guze SB. *Psychiatric Diagnosis*. 4th ed. New York, NY: Oxford University Press; 1989:22.

86. Goodwin DW, Preskorn SH. DSM-III and pharmacotherapy. In: Turner S, Hersen M, eds. *Adult Psychopathology: A Behavioral Perspective*. New York, NY: John Wiley & Sons; 1982:453-465.

87. Graber MA, Hoehns TB, Perry PJ. Sertraline-phenelzine drug interaction: a serotonin syndrome reaction. *Ann Pharmacother*. 1994;28:732-735.

88. Gram LF, Debruyne D, Caillard V, et al. Substantial rise in sparteine metabolic ratio during haloperidol treatment. *Br J Clin Pharmacol*. 1989;27:272-275.

89. Greb WH, Buscher G, Dierdorf HD, Koster FE, Wolf D, Mellows G. The effect of liver enzyme inhibition by cimetidine and enzyme induction by phenobarbitone on the pharmacokinetics of paroxetine. *Acta Psychiatr Scand*. 1989;350 (suppl):95-98.

90. Greist JH, Jefferson JW, Kobak KA, Katzelnick DJ, Serlin RC. Efficacy and tolerability of serotonin transport inhibitors in obsessive-compulsive disorder. A meta-analysis. *Arch Gen Psychiatry*. 1995;52:53-60.

91. Grimsley SR, Jann MW. Paroxetine, sertraline, and fluvoxamine: new selective serotonin reuptake inhibitors. *Clin Pharm*. 1992;11:930-957.

92. Harris MG, Benfield P. Fluoxetine. A review of its pharmacodynamic and pharmacokinetic properties, and therapeutic use in older patients with depressive illness. *Drugs Aging*. 1995;6:64-84.

93. Harvey AT, Preskorn SH. Cytochrome P450 enzymes: interpretation of their interactions with selective serotonin reuptake inhibitors. Part I. *J Clin Psychopharmacol*. 1996;16:273-285.

94. Harvey AT, Preskorn SH. Cytochrome P450 enzymes: interpretation of their interactions with selective serotonin reuptake inhibitors. Part II. *J Clin Psychopharmacol*. 1996;16:345-355.

95. Heinemann F, Assion HJ, Hermes G, Ehrlich M. Paroxetine-induced neuroleptic malignant syndrome [in German]. *Nervenarzt*. 1997;68:664-666.

96. Helzer JE, Burnam A, McEvoy LT. Alcohol abuse and dependence. In: Robins LN, Regier DA, Freedman DX, eds. *Psychiatric Disorders in America: The Epidemiological Catchment Area Study*. New York, NY: Free Press; 1991:81-115.

97. Heninger GR, Charney DS, Sternberg DE. Lithium carbonate augmentation of antidepressant treatment. An effective prescription for treatment-refactory depression. *Arch Gen Psychiatry*. 1983;40:1335-1342.

98. Hirschfeld RM, Keller MB, Panico S, et al. The National Depressive and Manic-Depressive Association consensus statement on the undertreatment of depression. *JAMA*. 1997;277: 333-340.

99. Holliday SM, Plosker GL. Paroxetine: a review of its pharmacology, therapeutic use in depression, and therapeutic potential in diabetic neuropathy. *Drugs Aging*. 1993;3:278-299.

100. Hutchinson DR, Tong S, Moon CA, Vince M, Clarke A. Paroxetine in the treatment of elderly depressed patients in general practice: a double-blind comparison with amitriptyline. *Int Clin Psychopharmacol*. 1992;6(suppl 4):43-51.

101. Hyttel J. Comparative pharmacology of selective serotonin reuptake inhibitors (SSRIs). *Nord J Psychiatry*. 1993;47(suppl 30):5-12.

102. Isaksen PM. The effect of an antidepressant agent on premature ejaculation [in Norwegian]. *Tidsskr Nor Laegeforen*. 1995;115:1616-1617.

103. Janicak PG, Davis JM, Preskorn SH, Ayd FJ Jr. *Principles and Practice of Psychopharmacotherapy*. 2nd ed. Baltimore, Md: Lippincott, Williams & Wilkins; 1997.

104. Jermain DM, Hughes PL, Follender AB. Potential fluoxetine-selegiline interaction. *Ann Pharmacother*. 1992;26:1300. Letter.

105. Joffe RT, Levitt AJ, Sokolov ST, Young LT. Response to an open trial of a second SSRI in major depression. *J Clin Psychiatry*. 1996;57:114-115.

106. Joffe RT, Singer W, Levitt AJ, et al. A placebo-controlled comparison of lithium and triidothyronine augmentation of tricyclic antidepressants in unipolar refractory depression. *Arch Gen Psychiatry*. 1993;50:387-393.

107. Kahn RS, Asnis GM, Wetzler S, van Praag HM. Neuroendocrine evidence for serotonin receptor hypersensitivity in panic disorder. *Psychopharmacology*. 1988;96:360-364.

108. Katona CL, Hunter BN, Bray J. A double-blind comparison of the efficacy and safety of paroxetine and imipramine in the treatment of depression with dementia. *Int J Geriatr Psychiatry*. 1998;13:100-108.

12

109. Kaul S, Shukla UA, Barbhaiya RH. Nonlinear pharmacokinetics of nefazodone after escalating single and multiple oral doses. *J Clin Pharmacol*. 1995;35:830-839.

110. Kaye CM, Haddock RE, Langley PF, et al. A review of the metabolism and pharmacokinetics of paroxetine in man. *Acta Psychiatr Scand*. 1989;350(suppl):60-75.

111. Kelland MD, Freeman AS, Chiodo LA. Serotonergic afferent regulation of the basic physiology and pharmacological responsiveness of nigrostriatal dopamine neurons. *J Pharmacol Exp Ther*. 1990;253:803-811.

112. Keller MB, Kocsis JH, Thase ME, et al. Maintenance phase efficacy of sertraline for chronic depression. A randomized controlled trial. *JAMA*. 1998;280:1665-1672.

113. Kerr JS, Fairweather DB, Mahendran R, Hindmarch I. The effects of paroxetine, alone and in combination with alcohol on psychomotor performance and cognitive function in the elderly. *Int Clin Psychopharmacol*. 1992;7:101-108.

114. Kessler LG, Cleary PD, Burke JD Jr. Psychiatric disorders in primary care. Results of a follow-up study. *Arch Gen Psychiatry*. 1985;42:583-587.

115. Ketter TA, Flockhart DA, Post RM, et al. The emerging role of cytochrome P450 3A in psychopharmacology. *J Clin Psychopharmacol*. 1995;15:387-398.

116. Kety SS. Genetic factors in suicide. In: Roy A, ed. *Suicide*. Baltimore, Md: Williams & Wilkins; 1986:41-45.

117. Keuthen NJ, Cyr P, Ricciardi JA, Minichiello WE, Buttolph ML, Jenike MA. Medication withdrawal symptoms in obsessive-compulsive disorder patients treated with paroxetine. *J Clin Psychopharmacol*. 1994;14: 206-207. Letter.

118. Kiloh LG, Andrews G, Neilson M. The long-term outcome of depressive illness. *Br J Psychiatry*. 1988;153:752-757.

119. Klamerus KJ, Maloney K, Rudolph RL, Sisenwine SF, Jusko WJ, Chiang ST. Introduction of a composite parameter to the pharmacokinetics of venlafaxine and its active O-desmethyl metabolite. *J Clin Pharmacol*. 1992;32:716-724.

120. Kline SS, Mauro LS, Scala-Barnett DM, Zick D. Serotonin syndrome versus neuroleptic malignant syndrome as a cause of death. *Clin Pharm*. 1989;8:510-514.

121. Knesper DJ, Riba MB, Schwenk TL. *Primary Care Psychiatry*. Philadelphia, Pa: WB Saunders Co; 1997.

122. Kupfer DJ. Long-term treatment of depression. *J Clin Psychiatry*. 1991;52(suppl):28-34.

123. Kupfer DJ, Frank E, Perel JM. Five-year outcome for maintenance therapies in recurrent depression. *Arch Gen Psychiatry*.1992;49:769-773.

124. Kupfer DJ, Frank E, Perel JM. The advantage of early treatment intervention in recurrent depression. *Arch Gen Psychiatry*.1989;46:771-775.

125. Landry P, Roy L. Withdrawal hypomania associated with paroxetine. *J Clin Psychopharmacol*. 1997;17:60-61.

126. Lazowick AL, Levin GM. Potential withdrawal syndrome associated with SSRI discontinuation. *Ann Pharmacother*. 1995;29:1284-1285.

127. Lebegue B. Mania precipitated by fluoxetine. *Am J Psychiatry*. 1987;144:1620. Letter.

128. Lejoyeux M, Ades J. Antidepressant discontinuation: a review of the literature. *J Clin Psychiatry*. 1997;58(suppl 7):11-16.

129. Leonard BE. The comparative pharmacology of new antidepressants [published erratum appears in *J Clin Psychiatry*. 1993;54:491]. *J Clin Psychiatry*. 1993;54(suppl):3-15.

130. Lewis J, Braganza J, Williams T. Psychomotor retardation and semistuporous state with paroxetine. *Br Med J*. 1993;306: 1169.

131. Lin KM, Poland RE. Ethnicity, culture and psychopharmacology. In: Bloom FE, Kupfer DJ, eds. *Psychopharmacology: The Fourth Generation of Progress*. New York, NY: Raven Press; 1994:1907-1918.

132. Liu B, Anderson G, Mittmann N, To T, Axcell T, Shear N. Use of selective serotonin-reuptake inhibitors or tricyclic antidepressants and risk of hip fractures in elderly people. *Lancet*. 1998;351:1303-1307.

133. Louie AK, Lannon RA, Ajari LJ. Withdrawal reaction after sertraline discontinuation. *Am J Psychiatry*. 1994;151:450-451. Letter.

134. Ludovico GM, Corvasce A, Pagliarulo G, Cirillo-Marucco E, Marano A, Pagliarulo A. Paroxetine in the treatment of premature ejaculation. *Br J Urol*. 1996;77:881-882.

135. Luvox (fluvoxamine maleate). *Compendium of Pharmaceuticals and Specialities*. 33rd ed. Ottawa, Ontario, Canada: Canadian Pharmaceutical Association; 1998;922-924.

136. Malek-Ahmadi P, Allen SA. Paroxetine-molindone interaction. *J Clin Psychiatry*. 1995;56:82-83. Letter.

137. Marshall RD, Schneier FR, Fallon BA, et al. An open trial of paroxetine in patients with noncombat-related, chronic posttraumatic stress disorder. *J Clin Psychopharmacol*. 1998;18:10-18.

138. Mathew NT, Tietjen GE, Lucker C. Serotonin syndrome complicating migraine pharmacotherapy. *Cephalalgia*. 1996;16: 323-327.

139. Mayol RF, Cole CA, Luke GM, Colson KL, Kerns EH. Characterization of the metabolites of the antidepressant drug nefazodone in human urine and plasma. *Drug Metab Dispos*. 1994;22:304-311.

140. McClelland GR, Raptopoulos P. Psychomotor effects of paroxetine and amitriptyline, alone and in combination with alcohol. *Br J Clin Pharmacol*. 1985;19:578P. Abstract.

141. McCombs JS, Nichol MB, Stimmel GL, Sclar DA, Beasley CM Jr, Gross LS. The cost of antidepressant drug therapy failure: a study of antidepressant use patterns in a Medicaid population. *J Clin Psychiatry*. 1990;51(suppl):60-69.

142. Merikangas KR, Weissman MM, Pauls DL. Genetic factors in the sex ratio of major depression. *Psychol Med*. 1985;15: 63-69.

143. Miller F, Friedman R, Tanenbaum J, Griffin A. Disseminated intravascular coagulation and acute myoglobinuric renal failure: a consequence of the serotonergic syndrome. *J Clin Psychopharmacol*. 1991;11:277-279. Letter.

144. Mills KC. Serotonin syndrome. *Am Fam Physician*. 1995;52:1475-1482.

145. Modell JG, Katholi CR, Modell JD, DePalma RL. Comparative sexual side effects of bupropion, fluoxetine, paroxetine, and sertraline. *Clin Pharmacol Ther*. 1997;61:476-487.

146. Montejo AI, Llorca G, Izquierdo JA, et al. Sexual dysfunction secondary to SSRIs. A comparative analysis in 308 patients [in Spanish]. *Actas Luso Esp Neurol Psiquiatr Cienc Afines*. 1996;24:311-321.

147. Montejo-Gonzales AL, Llorca G, Izquierdo JA, et al. SSRI-induced sexual dysfunction: fluoxetine, paroxetine, sertraline, and fluvoxamine in a prospective, multicenter, and descriptive clinical study of 344 patients. *J Sex Marital Ther*. 1997; 23:176-194.

148. Montgomery SA, Dufour H, Brion S, et al. The prophylactic efficacy of fluoxetine in unipolar depression. *Br J Psychiatry*. 1988;3(suppl):69-76.

149. Moreno FA, Geleberg AJ, Bachar K, Delgado PL. Pindolol augmentation of treatment-resistant depressed patients. *J Clin Psychiatry*. 1997;58:437-439.

150. Narayan M, Anderson G, Cellar J, Mallison RT, Price LH, Nelson JC. Serotonin transporter-blocking properties of nefazodone assessed by measurement of platelet serotonin. *J Clin Psychopharmacol*. 1998;18:67-71.

151. Nelson JC. Safety and tolerability of the new antidepressants. *J Clin Psychiatry*. 1997;58(suppl 6):26-31.

152. Nelson JC, Mazure CM. Lithium augmentation in psychotic depression refractory to combined drug treatment. *Am J Psychiatry*. 1986;143:363-366.

153. Nelson JC, Mazure CM, Bowers MB Jr, Jatlow PI. A preliminary, open study of the combination of fluoxetine and desipramine for rapid treatment of major depression. *Arch Gen Psychiatry*. 1991;48:303-307.

154. Neuvonen PJ, Pohjola-Sintonen S, Tacke U, Vuori E. Five fatal cases of serotonin syndrome after moclobemide-citalopram or moclobemide-clomipramine overdoses. *Lancet*. 1993;342;1419. Letter.

155. Nierenberg AA, Cole JO, Glass L. Possible trazodone potentiation of fluoxetine: a case series. *J Clin Psychiatry*. 1992;53:83-85.

156. Nierenberg AA, Feighner JP, Rudolph R, Cole JO, Sullivan J. Venlafaxine for treatment-resistant unipolar depression. *J Clin Psychopharmacol*. 1994;14:19-23.

157. Nierenberg AA, White K. What next? A review of pharmacologic strategies for treatment resistant depression. *Psychopharmacol Bull*. 1990;26:429-460.

158. Nierenberg DW, Semprebon M. The central nervous system serotonin syndrome. *Clin Pharmacol Ther*. 1993;53:84-88.

159. Oswald I, Adam K. Effects of paroxetine on human sleep. *Br J Clin Pharmacol*. 1986;22:97-99.

160. Parker G, Roy K, Hadzi-Pavlovic D, Pedic F. Psychotic (delusional) depression: a meta-analysis of physical treatments. *J Affect Disord*. 1992;24:17-24.

12

161. Paxil (paroxetine hydrochloride). In: *Physicians' Desk Reference*. 53rd ed. Montevale, NJ: Medical Economics Company, Inc; 1999:3078-3083.

162. Peet M. Induction of mania with selective serotonin re-uptake inhibitors and tricyclic antidepressants. *Br J Psychiatry*. 1994;164:549-550.

163. Pigott TA. OCD: where the serotonin selectivity story begins. *J Clin Psychiatry*. 1996;57(suppl 6):11-20.

164. Pincus HA, Tanielian TL, Marcus SC, et al. Prescribing trends in psychotropic medications: primary care, psychiatry, and other medical specialties. *JAMA*. 1998;279:526-531.

165. Pollock BG, Mulsant BH, Nebes R, et al. Serum anticholinergicity in elderly depressed patients treated with paroxetine or nortriptyline. *Am J Psychiatry*. 1998;155:1110-1112.

166. Potter WZ, Rudorfer MV, Manji H. The pharmacologic treatment of depression. *N Engl J Med*. 1991;325:633-642.

167. Preskorn S. Dose-effect and concentration-effect relationships with new antidepressants. In: Gram LF, Balant LP, Meltzer SG, Dahl SG, eds. *Clinical Pharmacology in Psychiatry: Strategies in Psychotropic Drug Development*. Berlin: Heidelberg; 1993:174-189.

168. Preskorn SH. A message from Titanic. *J Prac Psych Behav Hlth*. 1998;4:236-242.

169. Preskorn SH. Antidepressant drug selection: criteria and options. *J Clin Psychiatry*. 1994;55(suppl A):6-22, 23-24, 98-100.

170. Preskorn SH. *Clinical Pharmacology of Selective Serotonin Reuptake Inhibitors*. Caddo, Okla: Professional Communications, Inc; 1996.

171. Preskorn SH. Comparison of the tolerability of bupropion, fluoxetine, imipramine, nefazodone, paroxetine, sertraline, and venlafaxine. *J Clin Psychiatry*. 1995;56(suppl 6):12-21.

172. Preskorn SH. Debate resolved: there are differential effects of serotonin selective reuptake inhibitors on cytochrome P450 enzymes. *J Psychopharmacol*. 1998;12:S89-S97.

173. Preskorn SH. Do you feel lucky? *J Prac Psycho Behav Hlth*. 1998;4:37-40.

174. Preskorn SH. I don't see 'em. *J Prac Psych Behav Hlth*. 1997; 3:302-307.

175. Preskorn SH. Introduction: pharmacokinetics of psychotropic agents: why and how they are relevant to treatment. *J Clin Psychiatry*. 1993;54(suppl 9):3-7.

176. Preskorn SH. Pharmacokinetics of antidepressants: why and how they are relevant to treatment. *J Clin Psychiatry*. 1993;54 (suppl 9):14-34.

177. Preskorn SH. Recent dose-effect studies regarding antidepressants. In: Balant LP, Benitez J, Dahl SG, Gram LF, Pinder RM, Potter WZ, eds. *European Cooperation in the Field of Scientific and Technical Research*. Belguim: European Commission; 1998:45-61.

178. Preskorn SH. Selection of an antidepressant: mirtazapine. *J Clin Psychiatry*. 1997;58(suppl 6):3-8.

179. Preskorn SH. Serotonin receptor subtypes and their implications for psychiatric disorders. In: Hagerman RJ, McKenzie P, eds. *1992 International Fragile X Conference Proceedings*. Dillon, Colo: Spectra Publishing Co; 1992:179-194.

180. Preskorn SH. Should bupropion dosage be adjusted based upon therapeutic drug monitoring? *Psychopharmacol Bull*. 1991;27:637-643.

181. Preskorn SH. Should rational drug development in psychiatry target more than one mechanism of action in a single molecule? *Int Rev Psychiatry*. 1995;7:17-28.

182. Preskorn SH. The appearance of knowledge. *J Prac Psych Behav Hlth*. 1997;3:233-238.

183. Preskorn SH. The future and psychopharmacology: potentials and needs. *Psychiatr Ann*. 1990;20(suppl 11):625-633.

184. Preskorn SH. The revolution in psychiatry. *Phi Kappa Phi*. Winter 1993:22-25.

185. Preskorn SH. Tricyclic antidepressants: the whys and hows of therapeutic drug monitoring. *J Clin Psychiatry*. 1989;50 (suppl):34-42, 43-46.

186. Preskorn SH, Alderman J, Chung M, Harrison W, Messig M, Harris S. Pharmacokinetics of desipramine coadministered with sertraline or fluoxetine. *J Clin Psychopharmacol*. 1994;14:90-98.

187. Preskorn SH, Baker B. Fatality associated with combined fluoxetine-amitriptyline therapy. *JAMA*. 1997;277:1682. Letter.

12

188. Preskorn SH, Bupp S, Weller E, Weller R. Plasma levels of imipramine and metabolites in 68 hospitalized children. *J Am Acad Child Adoesc Psychiatry*. 1989;28:373-375.

189. Preskorn SH, Burke M. Somatic therapy for major depressive disorder: selection of an antidepressant. *J Clin Psychiatry*. 1992;53(suppl):5-18.

190. Preskorn SH, Fast GA. Beyond signs and symptoms: the case against a mixed anxiety and depression category. *J Clin Psychiatry*. 1993;54(suppl):24-32.

191. Preskorn SH, Fast GA. Therapeutic drug monitoring for antidepressants: efficacy, safety, and cost effectiveness [published erratum appears in *J Clin Psychiatry*. 1991;52:353]. *J Clin Psychiatry*. 1991;52(suppl):23-33.

192. Preskorn SH, Harvey A, Stanga C. Drug interactions and their role in patient care. *Curr Rev Mood Anxiety Disord*. 1997;1:203-214.

193. Preskorn SH, Jerkovich GS. Central nervous system toxicity of tricyclic antidepressants: phenomenology, course, risk factors, and the role of therapeutic drug monitoring. *J Clin Psychopharmacol*. 1990;10:88-95.

194. Preskorn SH, Kent TA. Mechanisms and interventions in tricyclic antidepressant overdoses. In: Stancer HC, Garfinkel PE, Rakoff VM, eds. *Guidelines for the Use of Psychotropic Drugs: A Clinical Handbook*. Spectrum Publications, Inc; 1984:63-75.

195. Preskorn SH, Lacey R. Polypharmacy: when is it rational? *J Prac Psych Behav Hlth*. 1995;1:92-98.

196. Preskorn SH, Othmer SC. Evaluation of bupropion hydrochloride: the first of a new class of atypical antidepressants. *Pharmacotherapy*. 1984;4:20-34.

197. Preskorn SH, Shad MU, Alderman J, Lane R. Fluoxetine: age and dose dependent pharmacokinetics and CYP 2C19 inhibition. *Am Soc Clin Pharmacol Ther*. 1998;63:166. Abstract.

198 Price JS, Waller PC, Wood SM, MacKay AV. A comparison of the post-marketing safety of four selective serotonin reuptake inhibitors including the investigation of symptoms occurring on withdrawal. *Br J Clin Pharmacol*. 1996;42:757-763.

199. Prien RF, Kupfer DJ. Continuation drug therapy for major depressive episodes: how long should it be maintained? *Am J Psychiatry*. 1986;143:18-23.

200. Prozac (fluoxetine hydrochloride). In: *Physicians' Desk Reference*. 53rd ed. Montvale, NJ: Medical Economics Company, Inc; 1999:924-928.

201. Quitkin FM, Harrison W, Liebowitz M, et al. Defining the boundaries of atypical depression. *J Clin Psychiatry*. 1984; 045:19-21.

202. Redux (dexfenfluramine hydrochloride) [package insert]. Philadelphia, Pa: Wyeth-Ayerst Laboratories; 1996.

203. Remeron (mirtazapine). In: *Physicians' Desk Reference*. 53rd ed. Montvale, NJ: Medical Economics Company, Inc: 1999:2147-2149.

204. Reynolds RD. Serotonin syndrome: what family physicians need to know. *Am Fam Physician*. 1995;52:1263, 1266, 1271. Editorial.

205. Robertson MM, Trimble MR. Depressive illness in patients with epilepsy: a review. *Epilepsia*. 1983;24(suppl 2):S109-S116.

206. Robins E. Completed suicide. In: Roy A, ed. *Suicide*. Baltimore, Md: Williams & Wilkins; 1986:123-133.

207. Robins E. *The Final Months: A Study of the Lives of 134 Persons Who Committed Suicide*. New York, NY: Oxford University Press; 1981.

208. Robinson DS, Roberts DL, Smith JM, et al. The safety profile of nefazodone. *J Clin Psychiatry*. 1996;57(suppl 2):31-38.

209. Rosenbaum JF, Fava M, Hoog SL, Ascroft RC, Krebs WB. Selective serotonin reuptake inhibitor discontinuation syndrome: a randomized clinical trial. *Biol Psychiatry*. 1998;44: 77-87.

210. Rosenbaum JF, Zajecka J. Clinical management of antidepressant discontinuation. *J Clin Psychiatry*. 1997;58(suppl 7):37-40.

211. Roth A, Akyol S, Nelson JC. Delirium associated with the combination of a neuroleptic, an SSRI, and benztropine. *J Clin Psychiatry*. 1994;55:492-495.

212. Rouillon F, Gorwood P. The use of lithium to augment antidepressant medication. *J Clin Psychiatry*. 1998;59(suppl 5):32-39.

12

213. Rowland DL, Myers L, Culver A, Davidson JM. Bupropion and sexual function: a placebo-controlled prospective study on diabetic men with erectile dysfunction. *J Clin Psychopharmacol.* 1997;17:350-357.

214. Rush AJ, Armitage R, Gillin JC, et al. Comparative effects of nefazodone and fluoxetine on sleep in outpatients with major depressive disorder. *Biol Psychiatry.* 1998;44:3-14.

215. Rush AJ, Kupfer DJ. Strategies and tactics in the treatment of depression. In: Gabbard GO, ed. *Treatments of Psychiatric Disorders.* 2nd ed. Washington, DC: American Psychiatric Press, Inc; 1996.

216. Sackeim HA, Devanand DP, Nobler MS. Electroconvulsive therapy. In: Bloom FE, Kupfer DJ, eds. *Psychopharmacology: The Fourth Generation of Progress.* New York, NY: Raven Press; 1994:1123-1142.

217. Saletu B, Frey R, Krupka M, Anderer P, Grünberger J, See WR. Sleep laboratory studies on the single-dose effects of serotonin reuptake inhibitors paroxetine and fluoxetine on human sleep and awakening qualities. *Sleep.* 1991;14:439-447.

218. Sanders-Bush E, Mayer SE. 5-Hydroxytryptamine (serotonin) receptor agonists and antagonists. In: Gilman AG, consulting ed; Hardman JG, Limbird LE, eds-in-chief; Molinoff PB, Ruddon RW, eds. *Goodman and Gilman's: The Pharmacological Basis of Therapeutics.* 9th ed. New York, NY: McGraw-Hill Book Co; 1996:249-266.

219. Schatzberg AF, Haddad P, Kaplan EM, et al. Possible biological mechanisms of the serotonin reuptake inhibitor discontinuation syndrome. Discontinuation Consensus Panel. *J Clin Psychiatry.* 1997;58(suppl 7):23-27.

220. Schwartz JC, Arrang JM, Garbarg M, Traiffort E. Histamine. In: Bloom FE, Kupfer DJ, eds. *Psychopharmacology: The Fourth Generation of Progress.* New York, NY: Raven Press; 1994;397-406.

221. Series HG. Drug treatment of depression in medically ill patients. *J Psychosom Res.* 1992;36:1-16.

222. Settle EC Jr, Settle GP. A case of mania associated with fluoxetine. *Am J Psychiatry.* 1984;141:280-281.

223. Shad MU, Preskorn SH. Antidepressants. In: Levy R, Thummel KE, Trager W, Hansten PD, Eichelbaum M, eds. *Metabolic Drug Interactions — Drugs as Inhibitors of Metabolic Enzymes Treatment of CNS Diseases.* Philadelphia, Pa: Lippincott, Williams & Wilkins. In press.

224. Shad MU, Preskorn SH. A drug-drug interaction in reverse: loss of phenytoin efficacy as a result of fluoxetine discontinuation. *J Clin Psychopharmacol.* In press. Letter.

225. Shad MU, Preskorn SH. A possible bupropion and imipramine interaction. *J Clin Psychopharmacol.* 1997;17:118-119. Letter.

226. Sharpley AL, Williamson DJ, Attenburrow ME, Pearson G, Sargent P, Cowen PJ. The effects of paroxetine and nefazodone on sleep: a placebo controlled trial. *Psychopharmacology.* 1996;126:50-54.

227. Spielberg SP. N-acetyltransferases: pharmacogenetics and clinical consequences of polymorphic drug metabolism. *J Pharmacokinet Biopharm.* 1996;24:509-519.

228. Sporer KA. The serotonin syndrome. Implicated drugs, pathophysiology and management. *Drug Saf.* 1995;13:94-104.

229. Stahl MM, Lindquist M, Pettersson M, et al. Withdrawal reactions with selective serotonin re-uptake inhibitors as reported to the WHO system. *Eur J Clin Pharmacol.* 1997;53:163-169.

230. Staner L, Kerkhofs M, Detroux D, Leyman S, Linkowski P, Mendlewicz J. Acute, subchronic and withdrawal sleep EEG changes during treatment with paroxetine and amitriptyline: a double-blind randomized trial in major depression. *Sleep.* 1995;18:470-477.

231. Stein G, Bernadt M. Lithium augmentation therapy in tricyclic-resistant depression. A controlled trial using lithium in low and normal doses. *Br J Psychiatry.* 1993;162:634-640.

232. Sternbach H. Danger of MAOI therapy after fluoxetine withdrawal. *Lancet.* 1988;2:850-851. Letter.

233. Sternbach H. The serotonin syndrome. *Am J Psychiatry.* 1991;148:705-713.

234. Stuppaeck CH, Geretsegger C, Whitworth AB, et al. A multicenter double-blind trial of paroxetine versus amitriptyline in depressed inpatients. *J Clin Psychopharmacol.* 1994;14:241-246.

235. Sussman N. Anxiolytic antidepressant augmentation. *J Clin Psychiatry*. 1998;59(suppl 5):42-48.

236. Tallman JF, Dahl SG. New drug design in psychopharmacology: the impact of molecular biology. In: Bloom FE, Kupfer DJ, eds. *Psychopharmacology: The Fourth Generation of Progress*. New York, NY: Raven Press; 1994:1861-1874.

237. Taylor DP, Carter RB, Eison AS, et al. Pharmacology and neurochemistry of nefazodone, a novel antidepressant drug. *J Clin Psychiatry*. 1995;56(suppl 6):3-11.

238. Tecott LH, Sun LM, Akana SF, et al. Eating disorder and epilepsy in mice lacking 5-HT2c serotonin receptors. *Nature*. 1995;374:542-546.

239. Thapa PB, Gideon P, Cost TW, Milam AB, Ray WA. Antidepressants and the risk of falls among nursing home residents. *N Engl J Med*. 1998;339:875-882.

240. Thase ME. Effects of venlafaxine on blood pressure: a meta-analysis of original data from 3744 depressed patients. *J Clin Psychiatry*. 1998;59:502-508.

241. Thase ME. The undertreatment of patients with depression. *Depressive Disorders: Index and Reviews*. 1996;1:4, 16-17.

242. Thase ME, Blomgren SL, Birkett MA, Apter JT, Tepner RG. Fluoxetine treatment of patients with major depressive disorder who failed initial treatment with sertraline. *J Clin Psychiatry*. 1997;58:16-21.

243. Thase ME, Frank E, Mallinger AG, Hamer T, Kupfer DJ. Treatment of imipramine-resistant recurrent depression, III: Efficacy of monoamine oxidase inhibitors. *J Clin Psychiatry*. 1992;53:5-11.

244. Thase ME, Howland RH, Friedman ES. Treating antidepressant nonresponders with augmentation strategies: an overview. *J Clin Psychiatry*. 1998;59(suppl 5):5-12, 13-15.

245. Thase ME, Rush AJ. Treatment-resistant depression. In: Bloom FE, Kupfer DJ, eds. *Psychopharmacology: The Fourth Generation of Progress*. New York, NY: Raven Press; 1994: 1081-1097.

246. Thase ME, Rush AJ. When at first you don't succeed: sequential strategies for antidepressant nonresponders. *J Clin Psychiatry*. 1997;58(suppl 13):23-29.

247. The APA Task Force on Laboratory Tests in Psychiatry. The dexamethasone suppression test: an overview of its current status in psychiatry. *Am J Psychiatry*. 1987;144:1253-1262.

248. Thomas DR, Nelson DR, Johnson AM. Biochemical effects of the antidepressant paroxetine, a specific 5-hydroxytryptamine uptake inhibitor. *Psychopharmacology*. 1987;93:193-200.

249. Tielens JA. Vitamin C for paroxetine- and fluvoxamine-associated bleeding. *Am J Psychiatry*. 1997;154:883-884. Letter.

250. Treatment of panic disorder. NIH Consensus Statement Online. 1991; September 25-27; 9(2):1-24.

251. Tucker P, Adamson P, Miranda R Jr, et al. Paroxetine increases heart rate variability in panic disorder. *J Clin Psychopharmacol*. 1997;17:370-376.

252. Turner SM, Jacob RG, Beidel DC, Griffin S. A second case of mania associated with fluoxetine. *Am J Psychiatry*. 1985;142: 274-275. Letter.

253. Vogel GW, Vogel F, McAbee RS, Thurmond AJ. Improvement of depression by REM sleep deprivation. New findings and a theory. *Arch Gen Psychiatry*. 1980;37:247-253.

254. von Moltke LL, Greenblatt DJ, Harmatz JS, Shader RI. Cytochromes in psychopharmacology. *J Clin Psychopharmacol*. 1994;14:1-4. Editorial.

255. von Moltke LL, Greenblatt DJ, Schmider J, Harmatz JS, Shader RI. Metabolism of drugs by cytochrome P450 3A isoforms. Implications for drug interactions in psychopharmacology. *Clin Pharmacokinet*. 1995;29(suppl 1):33-44.

256. Waldinger MD, Hengeveld MW, Zwinderman AH. Ejaculation-retarding properties of paroxetine in patients with primary premature ejaculation: a double-blind, randomized, dose-response study. *Br J Urol*. 1997;79:592-595.

257. Waldinger MD, Hengeveld MW, Zwinderman AH. Paroxetine treatment of premature ejaculation: a double-blind, randomized, placebo-controlled study. *Am J Psychiatry*. 1994:151:1377-1379.

258. Weilburg JB, Rosenbaum JF, Meltzer-Brody S, Shushtari J. Tricyclic augmentation of fluoxetine. *Ann Clin Psychiatry*. 1991;3:209-213.

259. Weissman MM. Affective disorders. In: Robins LN, Regier DA, eds. *Psychiatric Disorders in America: The Epidemiological Catchment Area Study*. New York, NY: Free Press; 1991:53-80.

260. Weissman MM, Klerman GL. Sex differences in the epidemiology of depression. *Arch Gen Psychiatry.* 1977;34:98-111.

261. Weissman MM, Leaf PJ, Holzer CE III, Myers JK, Tischler GL. The epidemiology of depression. An update on sex differences in rats. *J Affect Disord.* 1984;7:179-188.

262. Weissman MM, Wickramaratne P, Merikangas KR, et al. Onset of major depression in early adulthood. Increased familial loading and specificity. *Arch Gen Psychiatry.* 1984;41:1136-1143.

263. Weller EB, Weller RA, Fristad MA, Preskorn SH. The dexamethasone suppression test in hospitalized prepubertal depressed children. *Am J Psychiatry.* 1984;141:290-291.

264. Wells KB, Stewart A, Hays RD, et al. The functioning and well-being of depressed patients. Results from the Medical Outcomes Study. *JAMA.* 1989;262:914-919.

265. Wender PH. Pharmacotherapy of attention-deficit/hyperactivity disorder in adults. *J Clin Psychiatry.* 1998;59(suppl 7):76-79.

266. Wernicke JF. The side effect profile and safety of fluoxetine. *J Clin Psychiatry.* 1985;46:59-67.

267. Wheatley DP, van Moffaert M, Timmerman L, Kremer CM. Mirtazapine: efficacy and tolerability in comparison with fluoxetine in patients with moderate to severe major depressive disorder. Mirtazapine-Fluoxetine Study Group. *J Clin Psychiatry.* 1998;59:306-312.

268. Winokur G. Unipolar depression: is it divisible into autonomous subtypes? *Arch Gen Psychiatry.* 1979;36:47-52.

269. Winokur G, Tsuang MT, Crowe RR. The Iowa 500: affective disorder in relatives of manic and depressed patients. *Am J Psychiatry.* 1982;139:209-212.

270. Wolkenstein P, Cremniter D, Roujeau JC. Toxic epidermal necrolysis after paroxetine treatment. *Eur Psychiatry.* 1995;10:162. Letter.

271. Yocca FD, Hyslop DK, Taylor DP. Nefazodone: a potential broad spectrum antidepressant. *Trans Am Soc Neurochem.* 1985;16:115.

272. Zajecka J, Tracy KA, Mitchell S. Discontinuation symptoms after treatment with serotonin reuptake inhibitors: a literature review. *J Clin Psychiatry.* 1997;58:291-297.

273. Zoloft (sertraline hydrochloride). In: *Physicians' Desk Reference*. 53rd ed. Montvale, NJ: Medical Economics Company, Inc; 1999:2443-2448.

274. Zyban (bupropion hydrochloride). In: *Physicians' Desk Reference*. 53rd ed. Montvale, NJ: Medical Economics Company, Inc; 1999:1277-1282.

275. Zygmont M, Prigerson HG, Houck PR, et al. A post hoc comparison of paroxetine and nortriptyline for symptoms of traumatic grief. *J Clin Psychiatry*. 1998;59:241-245.

12

Note: Page numbers in *italics* indicate figures; page numbers followed by t indicate tables.

13

13

13

13

13

13

13

13

13

13

13

Propranolol (Inderal) B Blocker perform. anfiety
& muchused